Scented Candles

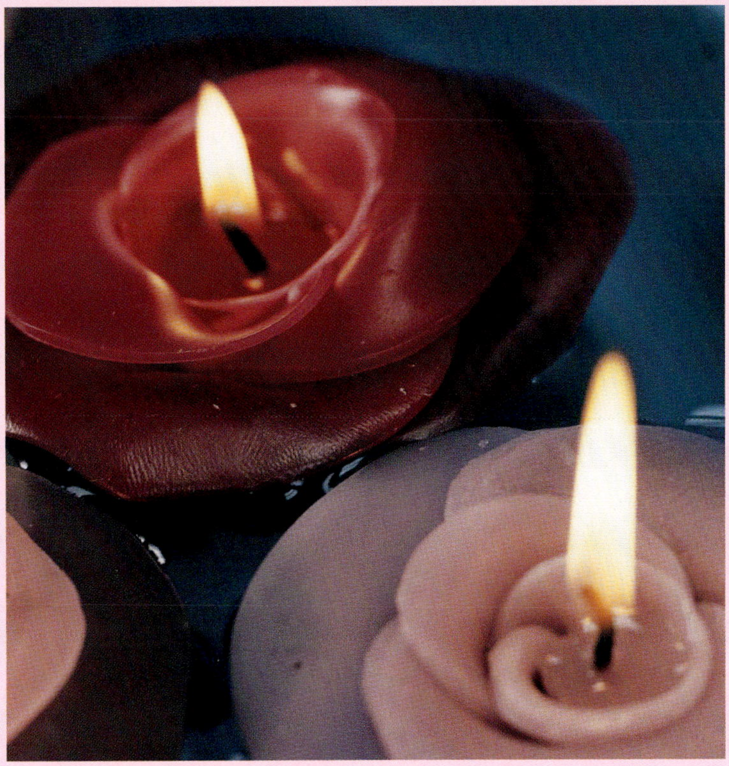

Scented Candles

20 FRAGRANT
PROJECTS
FOR ALL OCCASIONS

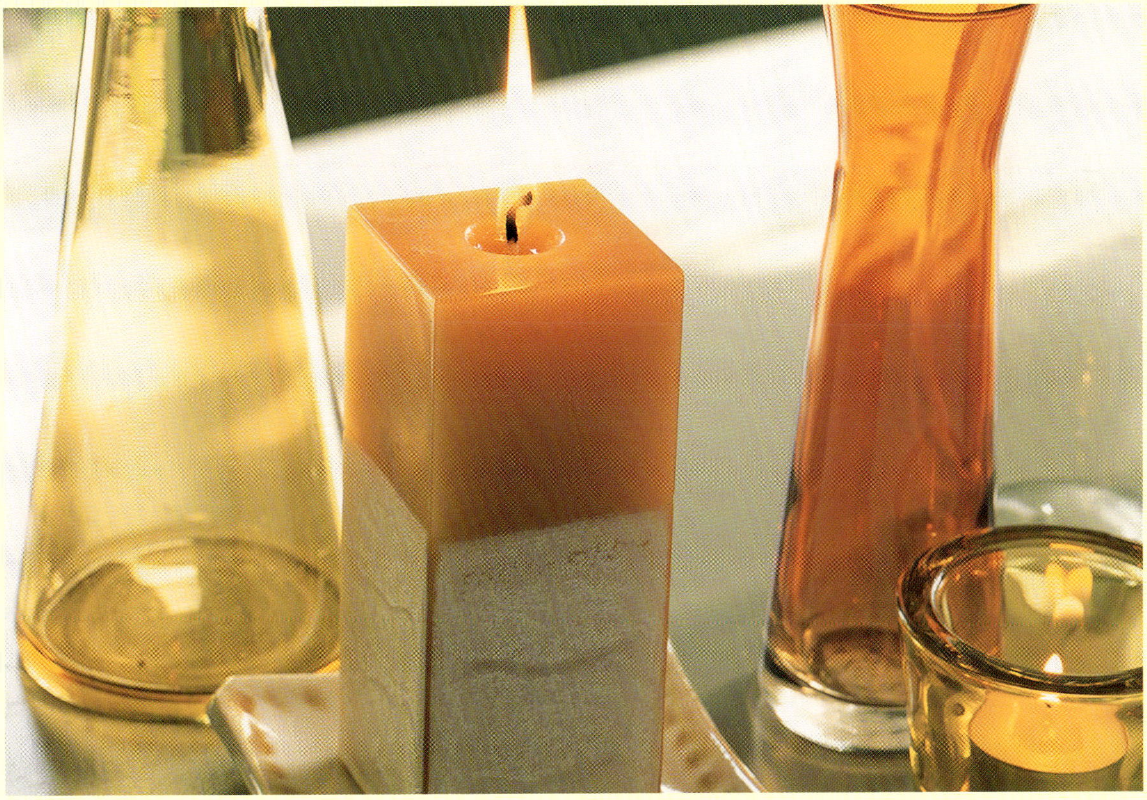

GLORIA NICOL

CICO BOOKS

London

The book is dedicated to my two brothers, Chris and Ken Nicol.

First published in 2003 by Cico Books Ltd
32 Great Sutton Street London EC1V 0NB

10 9 8 7 6 5 4 3 2 1

A CIP catalogue record for this book is available from the British Library

ISBN 1 903116 67 8

Editor: Gillian Haslam
Designer: Christine Wood
Photographer: Gloria Nicol

WARNING: CANDLES CAN CAUSE FIRE

Do not attempt any of the projects in this book without consulting the Perfume Safety and Using Candles Guidelines which are to be found in the Techniques section.

Please enjoy your candles by following these safety guidelines at all times:

Keep the wick on your candle trimmed to ⅛–¼-in. high. Never allow a candle to burn down to the bottom of its container. Do not allow a candle to burn for over 3 hours at a time. Always keep candles out of reach of pets, children, and away from polished surfaces, fabrics, drapes, and any flammable home furnishings. Never place a candle on an unstable surface and always keep it in a tray or safety container. If your candle contains free-floating items, then be sure to remove the pieces as the candle burns down. Use your common sense and exercise caution at all times.

If you are giving candles as gifts, do supply a copy of these safety guidelines to the recipient.

NEVER LEAVE A BURNING CANDLE UNATTENDED

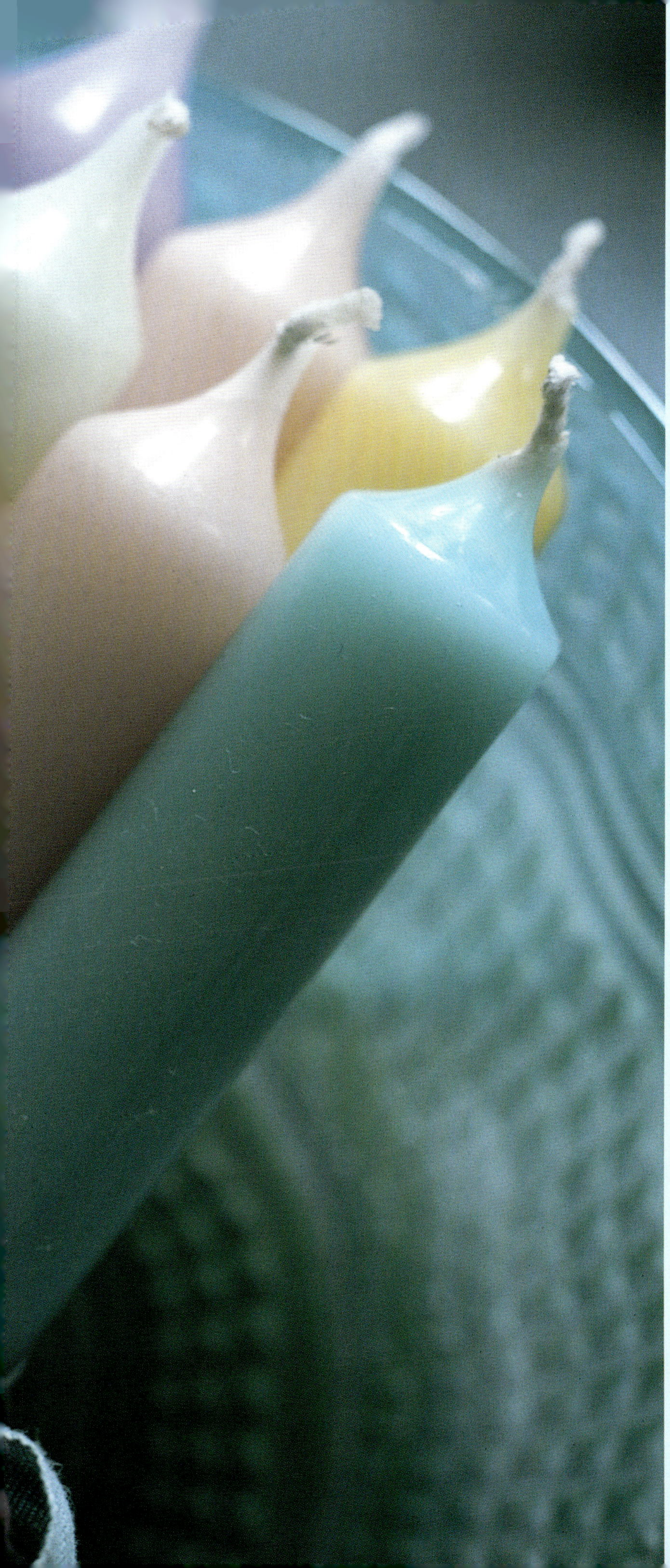

contents

introduction

From our first fond memories of blowing out the candles on a birthday cake, candlelight holds a special magic that weaves itself, like a continuous thread, through the achievements and celebrations throughout our lives. Candlelight has an exceptional quality that never seems to lose its mesmerizing attraction, and, whether it is simply a single candle glimmering in a glass bowl or a grand display of church candles in a cathedral adding to the spiritual ambience, it creates a special atmosphere. The ritual and ceremony of lit candles have a powerful and important significance. The increasing interest in aromatherapy and all things holistic is where candles really come into their own. When scented with essential oils and candle perfumes, candles can have a positive effect on how we live and the space we live in. By combining our own customized blends of scents, it is possible to alter the atmosphere in a room and create a feeling of wellbeing that particularly suits our own personal needs. They create a treat for the senses, can change the mood in the room, and have the potential to help us shake off the stresses of the day.

NOTE: The instructions in this book are given in imperial measurements. Use the conversion chart to work in metric, but do not change measurement systems within the project.

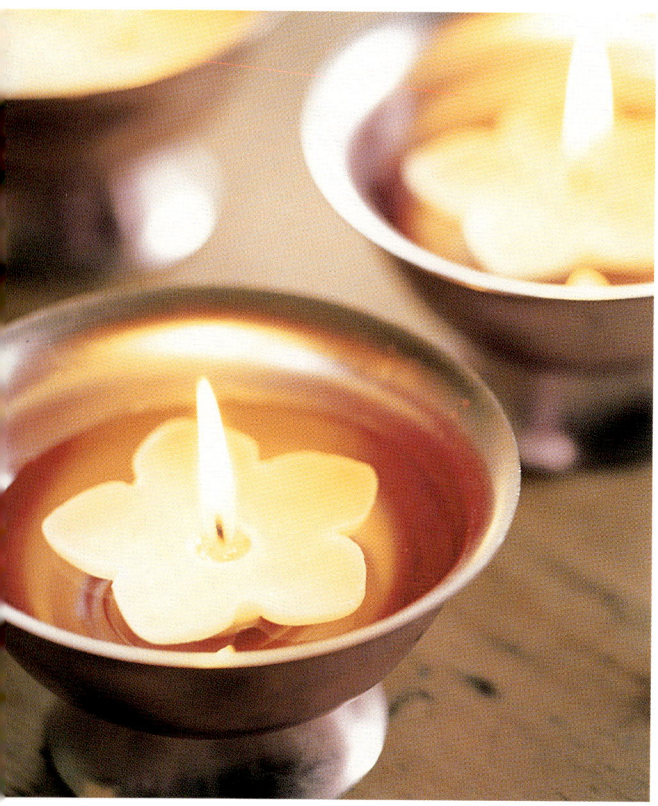

MEASUREMENTS

IMPERIAL to METRIC

⅛ in.	3 mm.	3 in.	7.5 cm.
¼ in.	6 mm.	4 in.	10 cm.
½ in.	13mm.	5 in.	12.5 cm
¾ in.	2 cm.	6 in.	15 cm.
1 in.	2.5 cm.	8 in.	20 cm.
1½ in.	4 cm.	12 in.	30 cm.
2 in.	5 cm.		

VOLUMES

IMPERIAL to METRIC

⅕ teaspoon	1 milliliter	1 fluid oz.	30 ml
1 oz.	28 grams	⅕ cup	47 ml
1 pound	454 grams	1 cup	237 ml
1 teaspoon	5 ml	1 pint	473 ml
1 tablespoon	15 ml		

TEMPERATURES

The instructions are given in Fahrenheit. To convert Fahrenheit to Celsius (Centigrade), use the ready reckoner right, or subtract 32 and divide by 1.8. Take care when heating wax, and always use a wax thermometer (see page 92).

FAHRENHEIT to CELSIUS

140 °F	60 °C
160 °F	71 °C
185 °F	85 °C
195 °F	90 °C
200 °F	93 °C
212 °F	100 °C
220 °F	104 °C

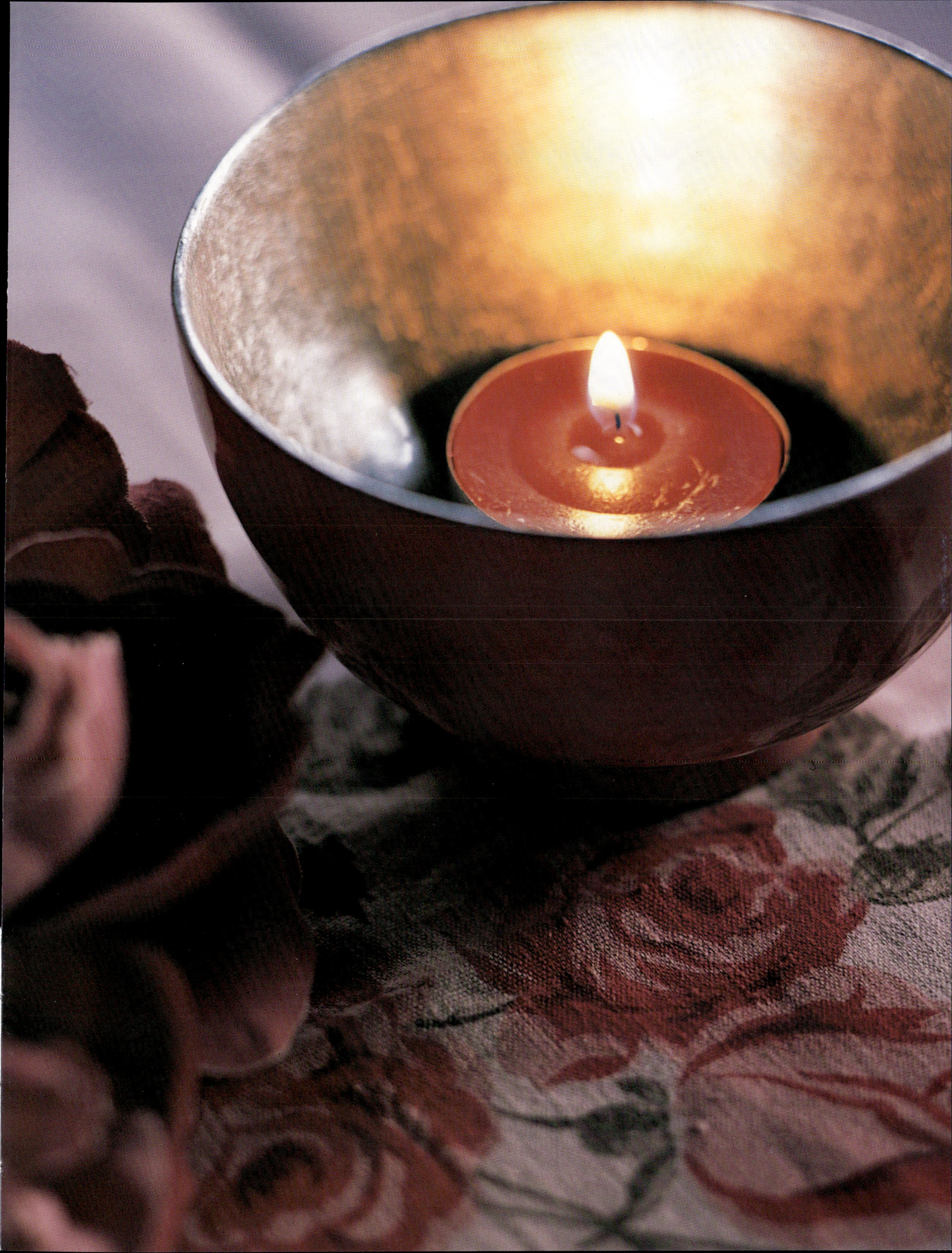

using essential oils

For centuries essential oils have been prized for their particular characteristics and magical abilities to encourage wellbeing, change moods, and heal ailments. They are extracted from the part of the plant that holds the scent—rose blooms give us their perfume; the unique aroma of geranium comes from the leaves; the roots of the plant produce the source of vetiver; oil and gum resins extracted from tree bark give us the essential scents of cedarwood, frankincense, and sandalwood. Some oils are less plentiful than others and consequently are more costly to buy. For example, pure rose oil—known as "rose otto" or "absolute"—requires 60,000 blooms to produce a mere ½ fl. oz. of precious oil. For candle making, there are many good synthetic perfumes available that are made especially for scenting wax, so it would be advisable in this instance to opt for the synthetic version. Candle perfumes are oil-soluble and specially formulated to be burned. The best of these contain natural flower and fruit essences.

From the hundreds of oils available, not all are suitable for scenting candles, either from a sensory perspective or a technical point of view. Oils can smell differently when they burn—sometimes not particularly pleasant or emit no scent at all—while some don't blend with wax or can leach out of the candle within days of making. It is important to do a couple of simple tests to check the suitability of the oils you choose for candle making before embarking on your projects.

THE SNIFF TEST

To test the scent, dip a strip of blotting paper, a paper spill, or a length of wick into the oil, then light it with a match and blow out the flame. Waft the smoke given off under your nose to get an accurate guide of the aroma it will produce in burning wax.

THE MIXING TEST

To test whether the oil will be suitable to combine with wax, melt approximately 1 oz. of wax in the top of a double boiler, heating to 180°F, and add 20 drops of oil. Pour the mixture into a ramekin and allow it to set. If the oil separates out of the wax, it will not be suitable for making candles.

COMBINING SCENTS

Blending scents is an art that requires skill and a keen nose. Essential oils vary in strength and evaporate at different rates, so they are perceived by our olfactory senses in a particular order. This scale of evaporation is divided into three parts: top notes, middle notes, and base notes. The top note is the scent you first become aware of when smelling a perfume. The middle notes come from the heart of the blend and the base notes provide the underlying layer that fixes the scent and makes it last. The desired result should be balanced with no single scent predominating. For a basic combination, try the aromatherapists' trick of clutching open bottles of oil together in one hand and circling them under your nose to give an approximation of how the fragrances will blend. Or employ the perfumiers' technique of using narrow strips of blotting paper to make absorbent spills and adding drops of different oils to each one, with more drops of lighter perfumes and less of the stronger ones. Sniff the spills in different combinations to find the mixtures you like best, trusting your instincts, and going for the scents that are your favorites.

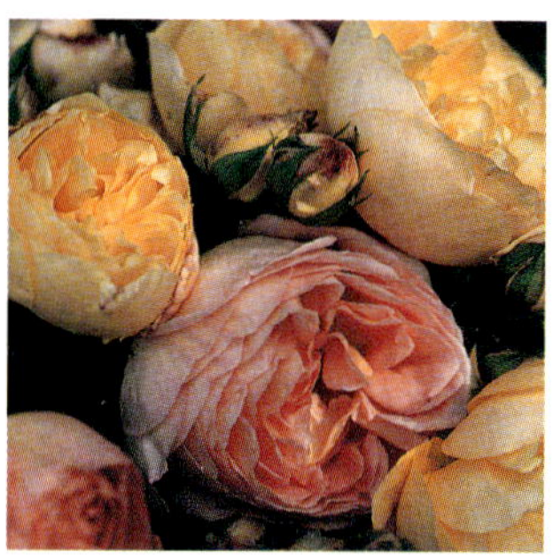

FLORAL

chamomile (anthemis nobilis)

Perfume note—middle. A soothing, calming, and relaxing oil that blends well with rosemary, lavender, jasmine, neroli, and bergamot.

jasmine (jasminum officinalis)

Perfume note—base. Jasmine is a particularly intense and heady scent that blends well with other floral fragrances and has uplifting and balancing characteristics. It is also reputed to possess aphrodisiac qualities. Try combinations with bergamot, orange, sandalwood, rose, and ylang-ylang.

lavender (lavandula angustifolia)
Perfume note—middle to top. Undoubtedly the most versatile oil of them all. Calming, balancing, and soothing, lavender has been used for centuries to encourage peaceful sleep. Blends well with citrus and floral oils including rose, bergamot, geranium, rosemary, patchouli, rose, and jasmine.

neroli (citrus aurantium)
Perfume note—middle. One of the most beautiful, luxurious floral oils when blended with other heady florals like rose absolute, jasmine absolute, and ylang-ylang. Stimulating, balancing, and uplifting, this oil also combines well with citrus oils.

rose (rosa damascena)
Perfume note—middle. Rose oil has an unmistakably rich and sweet floral scent that is extremely popular and classic. It can alleviate depression and is relaxing and uplifting. It blends with most oils, especially lavender, patchouli, sandalwood, ylang-ylang, and bergamot.

ylang-ylang (cananga odorata)
Perfume note—base to middle. A powerful, sweet, exotic scent with a balsamic undertone. Ylang-ylang is well known for its aphrodisiac qualities and can induce euphoria as well as being a natural sedative and antidepressant. The oil becomes more powerful when blended with other oils, and bergamot, jasmine, lemon, lavender, rose, rosewood, and sandalwood are particularly good choices.

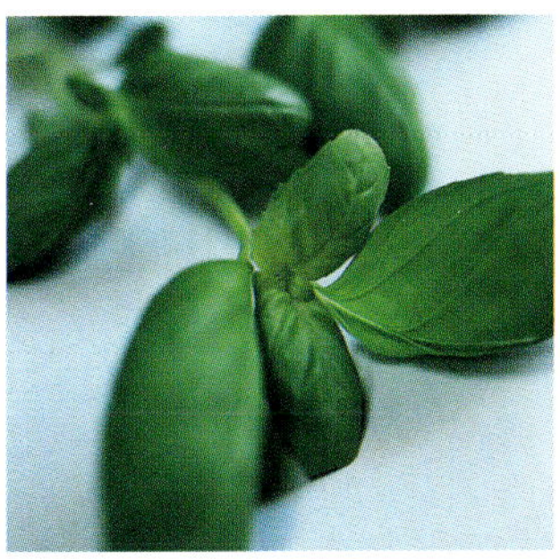

HERBAL

basil (ocimum basilicum)
Perfume note—top. Basil oil is strongly aromatic with a sweet licorice-like fragrance alongside an underlying hint of cloves. Invigorating and refreshing, it also has cooling, balancing, and restorative qualities. Basil oil works well with lavender, bergamot, black pepper, geranium, marjoram, and neroli.

geranium (pelargonium graveolens)
Perfume note—middle to top. A fresh, floral, and sweet-smelling oil that restores and stabilizes the emotions. Balancing and soothing. Combines well with lavender, bergamot, cedarwood, jasmine, lime, neroli, rose, rosemary, and sandalwood.

marjoram (origanum marjorana)
Perfume note—middle. Soothing, comforting, and warming, marjoram was thought by the ancient Greeks to bring good fortune and promote longevity. Blend with cedarwood, chamomile, lavender, mandarin, orange, nutmeg, rosemary, and ylang-ylang.

peppermint (mentha piperita)
Perfume note—top. Peppermint is usually used to give a lift to a blend. It is cool and fresh, and restores and uplifts with its energizing and stimulating properties. Has a special affinity with lavender and blends well with citrus oils as well as geranium, marjoram, rosemary, and sandalwood.

rosemary (rosmarinus officinalis)
Perfume note—middle. A distinctive and penetrating scent with clean, piney notes. Has stimulating, warming, strengthening, and reviving properties. Combines well with lavender, bergamot, basil, and all the citrus oils.

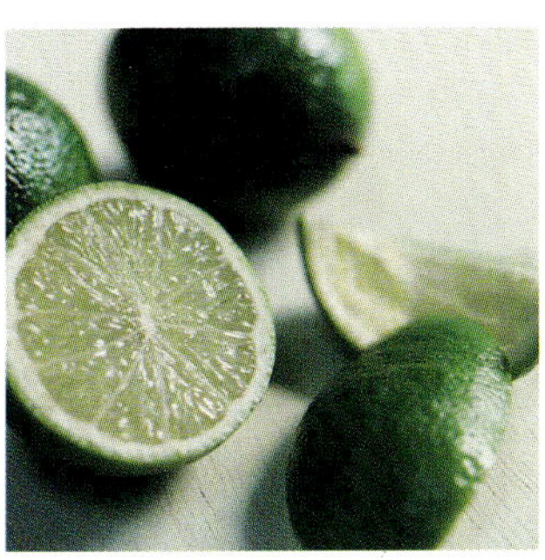

FRUITY

bergamot (citrus bergamia)
Perfume note—top. A cooling, calming, and uplifting fragrance that is said to be an anti-depressant. Blends well with chamomile, geranium, lavender, rosemary, neroli, and ylang-ylang.

citronella (cymbopogon nardus)
Perfume note—top. Used to scent outdoor candles to discourage mosquitoes.

grapefruit (citrus paradisi)
Perfume note—top. Grapefruit has a lovely, fresh aroma that cools and stimulates and is

refreshing and energizing. Blends with other citrus oils, especially bergamot and orange, as well as clove, ginger, lavender, rosemary, and other spices.

lemon citrus (limonium)
Perfume note—top. Lemon oil is antiseptic, cleansing, and stimulating. This versatile and energizing oil blends well with other citrus oils as well as lavender, ylang-ylang, geranium, neroli, sandalwood, and frankincense.

lime (citrus aurantiifolia)
Perfume note—top. Extracted from the fruit peels of limes from the West Indies, it acts like lemon and other citrus oils. Energizing and uplifting, mix lime with citronella, lavender, neroli, rosemary, mandarin, and basil.

mandarin (citrus reticulata)
Perfume note—top. A gentle and calming oil, mandarin is soothing and sedative. Mix with other citrus oils and spices such as bergamot and grapefruit, and floral scents like chamomile, geranium, lavender, neroli, and rose.

orange (citrus sinensis)
Perfume note—top. The rich, golden oil of sweet orange is a wonderful winter oil. It uplifts the spirits and is balancing and relaxing. Blends particularly well with spice oils and other citrus oils as well as geranium, lavender, myrrh, neroli, chamomile, and rosemary.

vanilla (vanilla planifolia)
Perfume note—base to middle. Not available as an essential oil but is extracted for a rich, full-bodied scent that acts as a bridge between other perfumes. Benzoin is the nearest oil with a similar fragrance and is sometimes used as a substitute for this highly popular fragrance. Blends well with other fruit and floral scents.

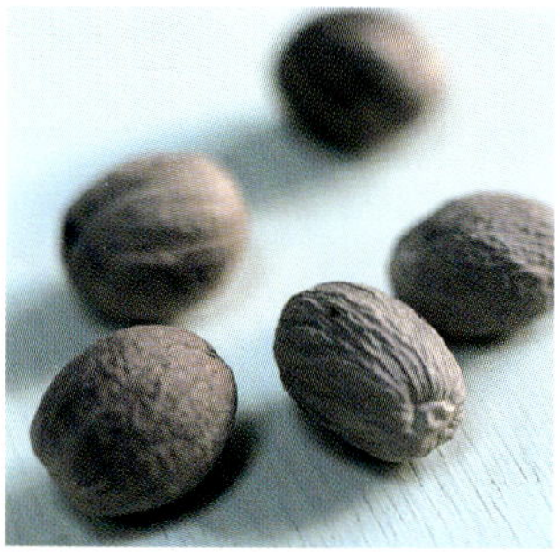

SPICY

black pepper (piper nigrum)
Perfume note—middle. Black pepper has a warm, dry, woody note with the ability to stimulate and tone. Also has aphrodisiac qualities. Combine with lavender, rose, rosemary, marjoram, sandalwood, and frankincense.

cardamom (elettaria cardamomum)
Perfume note—top. An intensely aromatic oil that is very pleasant, warm, and spicy with uplifting qualities. Also said to clear the mind. Blend with frankincense, geranium, ylang-ylang, rose, bergamot, lemon, and clove. Very pungent so use sparingly.

cinnamon (cinnamomum zeylanicum)
Perfume note—middle. Warm and sweetly spicy, cinnamon is uplifting and stimulating. Cinnamon blends well with citrus oils, clove, nutmeg, and frankincense.

clove (syzygium aromaticum syn. eugenia caryophyllata)
Perfume note—middle. Strong and fresh, this spicy aroma is stimulating and warming. Blends well with other spicy fragrances such as black pepper, nutmeg, and cinnamon as well as citronella, grapefruit, peppermint, basil, rosemary, and rose.

ginger (zingiber officinale)
Perfume note—top. A hot, spicy, pungent, and sweet-smelling oil. Ginger is energizing and stimulating, and is reputed to be an aphrodisiac. Blends well with cinnamon, frankincense, geranium, rose, and citrus oils such as lemon and lime.

nutmeg (myristica fragrans)
Perfume note—middle. Nutmeg has a warming scent and promotes restful sleep with dreams, and is also useful to counterbalance stress and tiredness. It blends well with bay, orange, geranium, rosemary, lime, petitgrain, and mandarin.

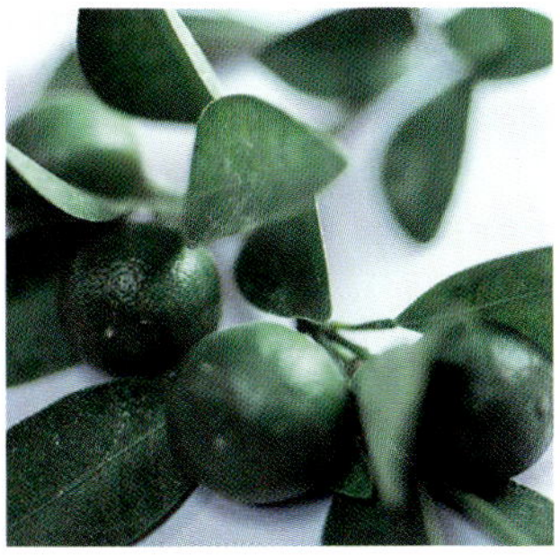

LEAFY

patchouli (pogostemon cablin syn. p.patchouli)

Perfume note—base. A distinctive and intensely fragranced oil that is an antidepressant, with sensual and soothing as well as stimulating properties. Blends with vetiver, sandalwood, cedarwood, geranium, clove, lavender, rose, neroli, bergamot, and myrrh.

petitgrain (citrus aurantium)

Perfume note—top. Another oil from the same tree as neroli and orange blossom. Petitgrain has a fresh, light, flowery perfume and is uplifting, revitalizing, and restoring. Blends well with rosemary, lavender, geranium, and bergamot.

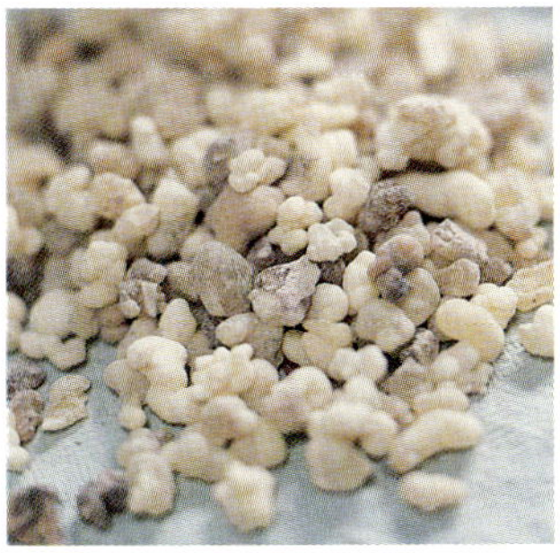

RESINOUS

benzoin (styrax benzoin)

Perfume note—base. A versatile sweet, balsamic scent reminiscent of vanilla. Blends equally well with floral and spice blends.

frankincense (boswellia thurifera)

Perfume note—base. Frankincense is known as olibanum and has soothing and warming characteristics. Used for centuries to burn on alters and in temples to create a spiritual atmosphere. Blends well with basil, black pepper, geranium, grapefruit, lavender, orange, patchouli, and sandalwood.

myrrh (commiphora myrrha)

Perfume note—base. Myrrh has a musty, slightly bitter scent that is toning, stimulating, and soothing. Creates a heavenly scent when burned together with frankincense. Other possible combinations include lavender, patchouli, and sandalwood.

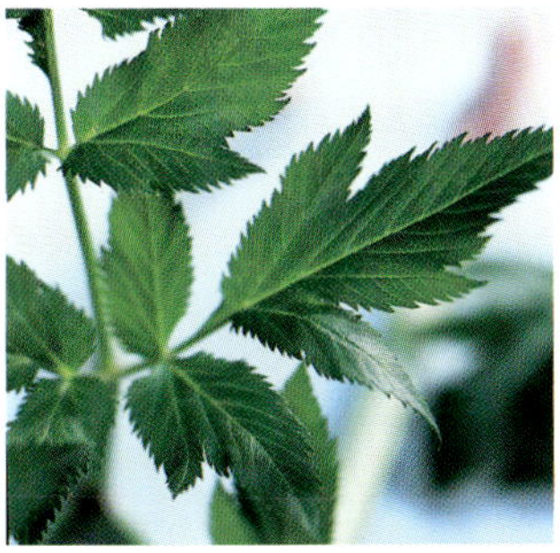

ROOTS

angelica (angelica archangelica)

Perfume note—base to middle. A warm, earthy aroma that is anchoring, restorative, and strengthening. Only a small quantity is needed to create an effect. Blends well with patchouli, frankincense, and citrus oils.

vetiver (vetiveria zizanioides)

Perfume note—base. A sweet, heavy, earthy aroma that is soothing, rejuvenating, and uplifting. Blends well with other natural antidepressant oils such as clary sage, jasmine, patchouli, lavender, rose, sandalwood, and ylang-ylang.

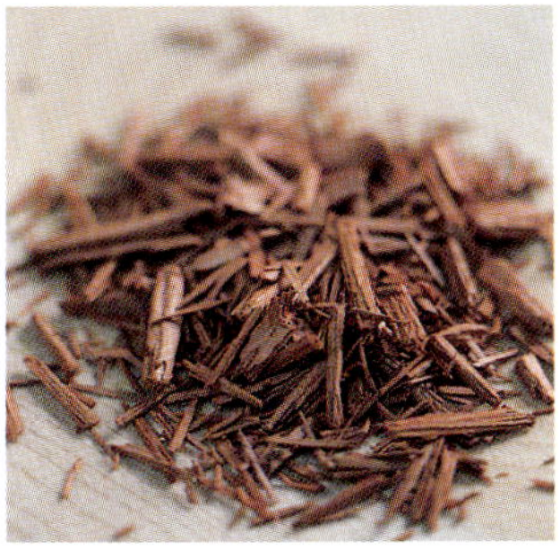

WOODY

cedarwood (cedrus atlantica)

Perfume note—base. Warm and woody, cedarwood soothes and harmonizes and is reputedly balancing and grounding. Combine with patchouli, vetiver, or sandalwood.

rosewood (aniba roseaodora)

Perfume note—middle to top. Known as an antidepressant, rosewood wards off general malaise and is deeply relaxing without being sedative; steadying and balancing. Combine with bergamot, cedarwood, clove, rose, frankincense, lemon, mandarin, and sandalwood.

sandalwood (santalum album)

Perfume note—base. A rich, exotic oil with a musky scent. Also has persistency and staying power. Reputedly an aphrodisiac, it has calming and grounding qualities. Blends well with rose, violet, clove, lavender, black pepper, bergamot, geranium, vetiver, patchouli, myrrh, and jasmine.

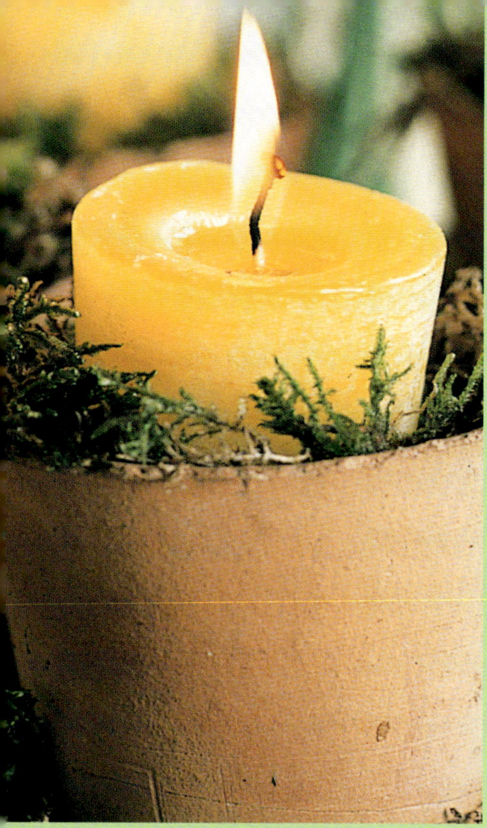

ESSENCE·OF spring

Spring is a time for new beginnings, revived optimism, and a fresh approach to the challenges of the year ahead. As the blooms of the season wait eagerly for just the right moment to burst into life, the horticultural year awakens from dormancy and begins its new cycle. To cherish and embrace these qualities for as long as possible, decorate and fragrance your home with the natural elements and fresh scents that are abundant at this time.

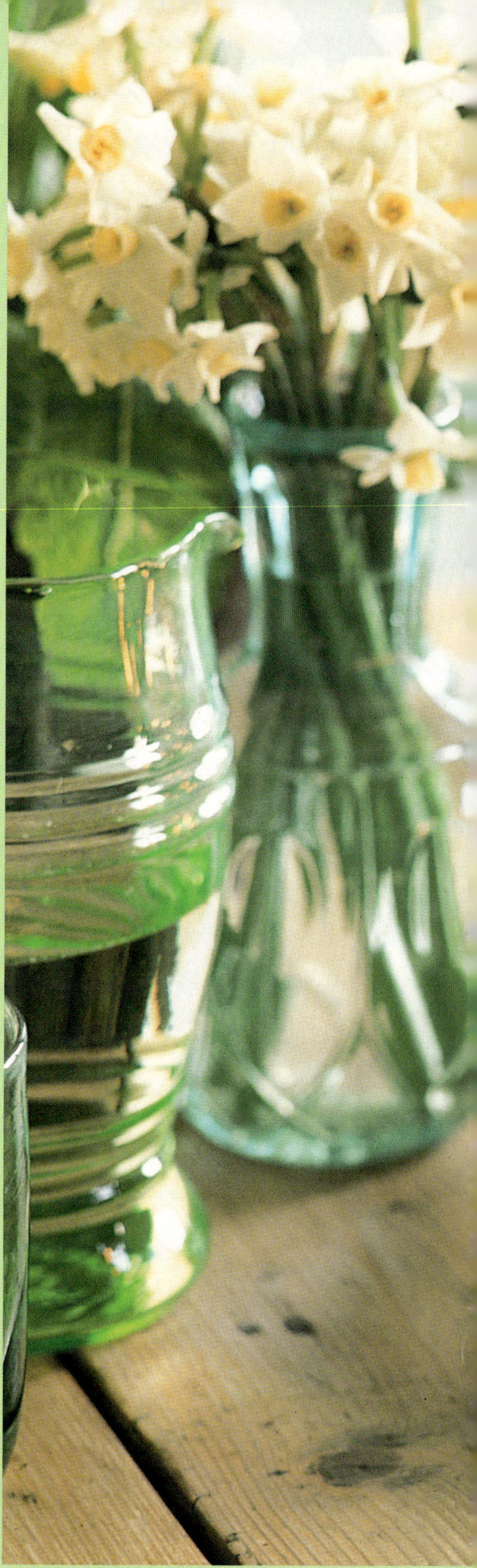

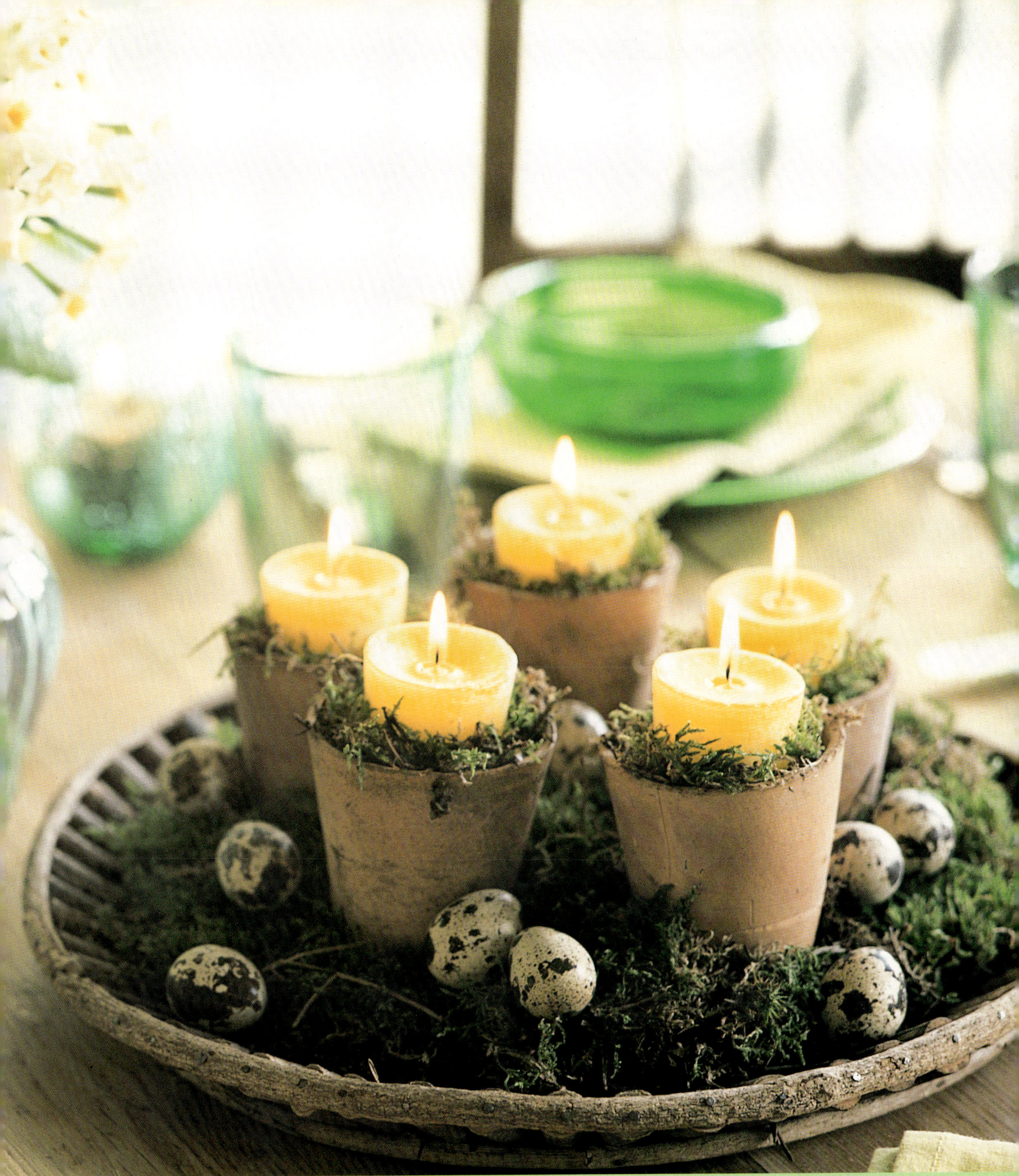

A table decorated with spring flowers and vibrant green moss brings the outdoors inside in celebration of the season, with the fabulous fresh scents of lime and cedar to invigorate those gathered around the table.

White flower scents have a universal appeal. These flowers—which include jasmine, ylang-ylang, gardenia, and tuberose—have been prized for centuries for their exquisite perfumes and mood-enhancing qualities. A classic cream-colored candle, set in a straight-sided glass, is the simplest to make, with one essential oil added to the molten wax. Just as a single gardenia bloom can scent an entire room, this glass container candle can re-create the ambience of an exotic garden and fill the room with its heady scent. Choose jasmine to create a relaxing and joyful atmosphere, ylang-ylang for a soothing and sensual mood, or tuberose for its reputed exotic and aphrodisiac qualities.

container candle

you will need:

Prepared medium container wick
Wick sustainer
Glass tumbler
8 oz. paraffin wax beads or beeswax (or a mixture of both)
Approximately 2 tsp. essential oil or candle perfume

MAKING THE CANDLE Slightly off-white wax looks far more stylish than bright white wax, so combine some natural honey-colored beeswax with the paraffin wax. You can recycle old beeswax candles (with the wicks removed) in this way. Beeswax also helps to prolong the burning time of the candle. Alternatively, add the tiniest amount of brown wax-soluble dye to the molten wax, but err on the side of caution. This glass tumbler is 3 inches in diameter and 4 inches tall, including the base.

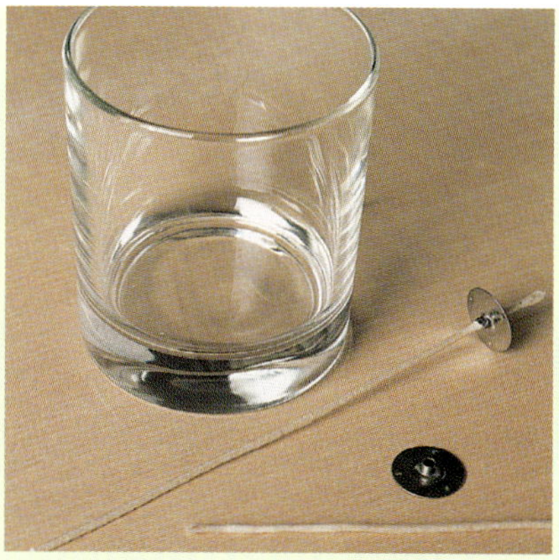

1 Cut the wick to the overall depth of the glass plus an extra inch. Thread the end of the wick through a wick sustainer. Close the metal hole around the wick with pliers to secure, then trim the end of the wick close to the base of the sustainer.

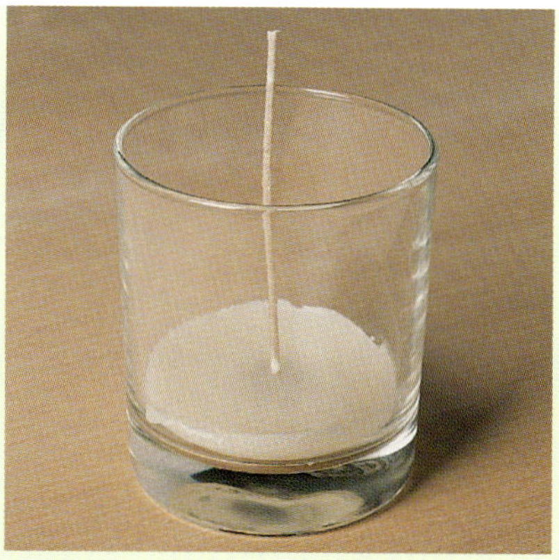

2 Melt the wax and heat to 180°F, then allow to cool slightly before adding the essential oil. Pour a tiny amount of molten wax into the glass to cover the base. Just as it begins to skin over, place the wick with sustainer into the center. Allow the wax to set.

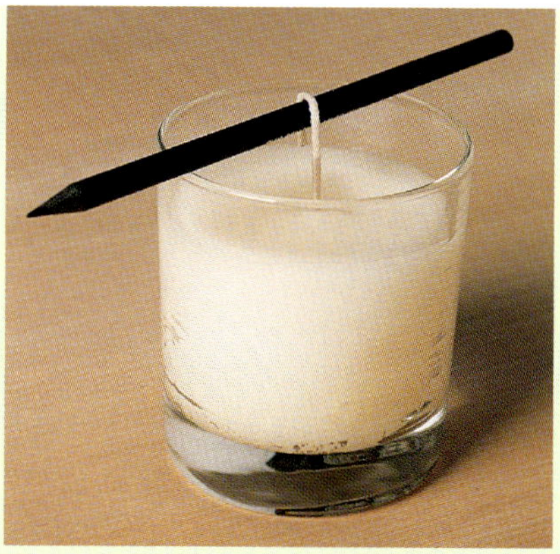

3 Wrap the excess wick around a pencil or wicking needle to hold it up straight in the glass. Reheat the wax to 180°F and carefully pour it into the glass, taking great care to prevent splashes around the rim. If the glass has a thick base, fill it with wax so the space below the rim matches the depth of the base. Allow to set.

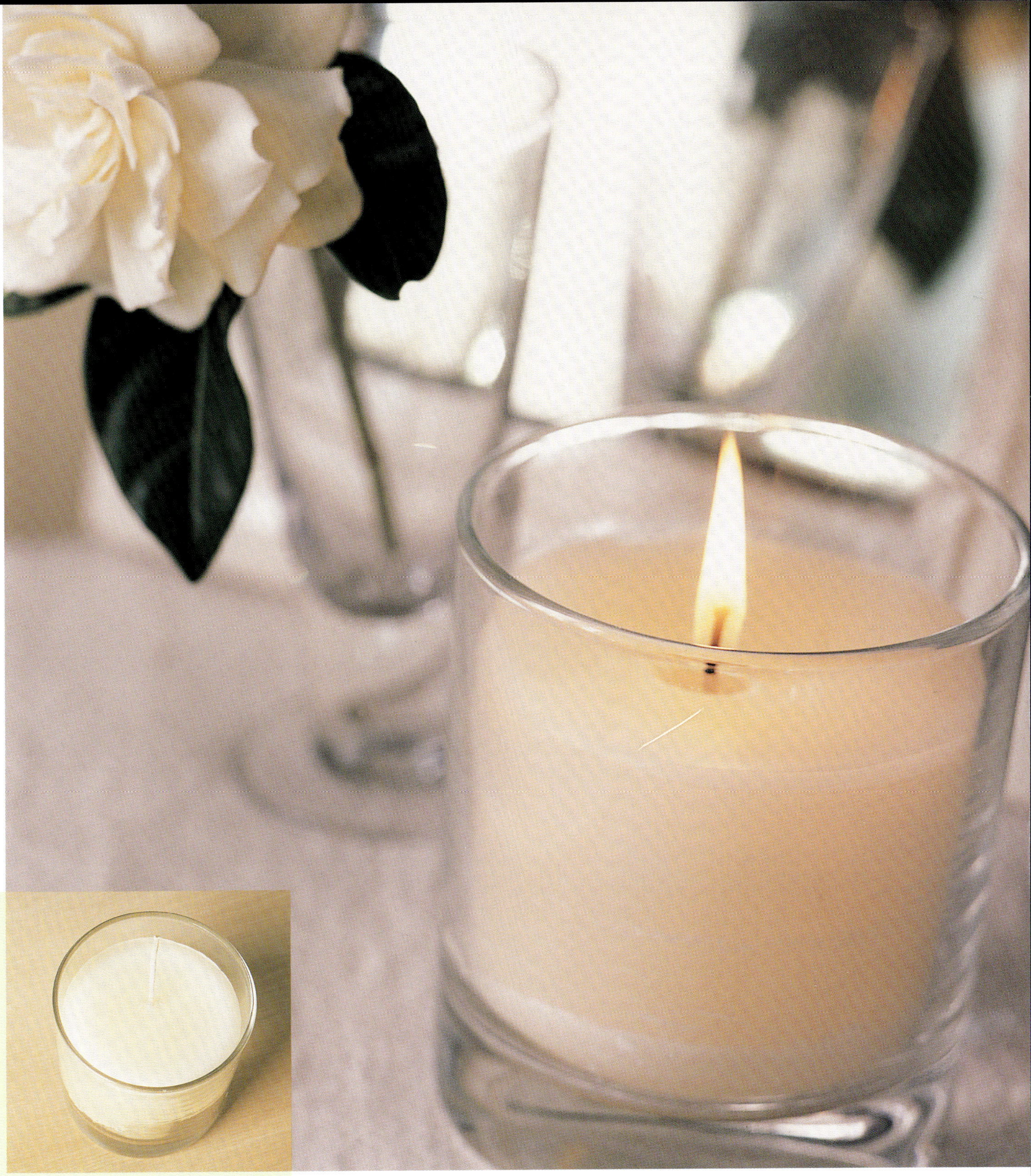

4 Pour more molten wax into the dip that forms as the wax sets and shrinks down around the wick, filling it level with the outer edge. Allow to set, then remove the pencil and trim the wick to size.

Use natural elements and fresh scents to decorate the table for a special meal. Lime-colored candles complement the bright yellows and fresh greens of spring flowers, wedged into terra-cotta pots with carpet moss around each rim. Arranged on a platter decked with more moss, real quails' eggs nestle among the pots to make a decorative as well as edible starter. The uplifting, positive fragrance of lime oil is reputed to be an appetite stimulant, while a dash of cedarwood brings an underlying woody note and a balancing partnership.

molded pillar candles

you will need (to make 1 candle):

Prepared medium wick
Wick sustainer
Small cylindrical molds
¼ oz. stearin
Wax dye
4 oz. paraffin wax beads
Approximately 1 tsp. essential oil or wax perfume

MAKING THE CANDLE Using small molds from the kitchen to make these candles rather than buying special candle molds is not only a less expensive option, but it also means you can make candles in batches. When choosing alternative molds, remember that the shape must be slightly wider at the top than at the base so the candle will slide out easily. Pouring the wax into the molds at a lower temperature will give an interesting textured surface. These candles have been colored to complement the other bright yellows and sharp greens in the arrangement, as well as matching the fruity scent. When using scents around food, it is important that there is nothing overpowering or conflicting between the perfumes and the aroma of the food. A good size mold would be 2½ inches across the base and 2½ inches tall.

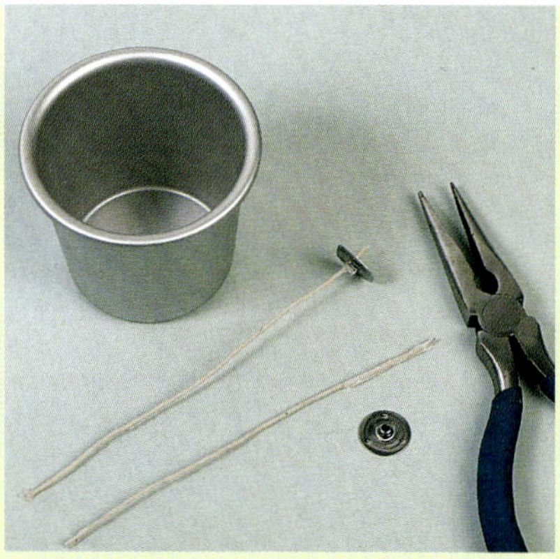

1 Cut the wick slightly longer than the height of the mold and attach a wick sustainer to one end using long-nosed pliers. With the sustainer resting on the mold's base, place the wick centrally in the mold and wind the excess wick around a wicking needle resting across the rim of the mold. Hold the needle in place with a piece of masking tape.

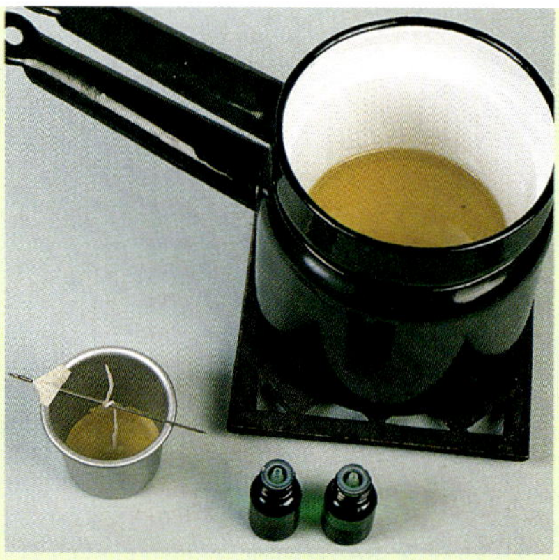

2 Melt the stearin and wax dye together, then add the paraffin wax and heat till completely melted. Stir in a few drops of oil or perfume, then pour a tiny amount of wax into the base of the mold to fix the wick in position. Allow to almost set.

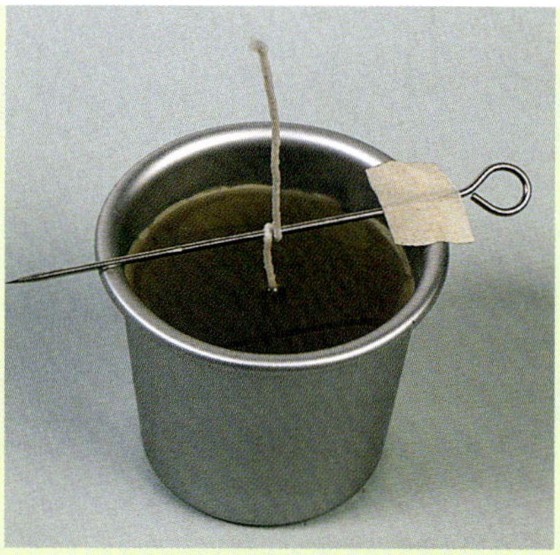

3 Heat the wax to 160°F and pour into the mold, almost to the top. Allow to set, weighed down in a water bath to help it cool more quickly.

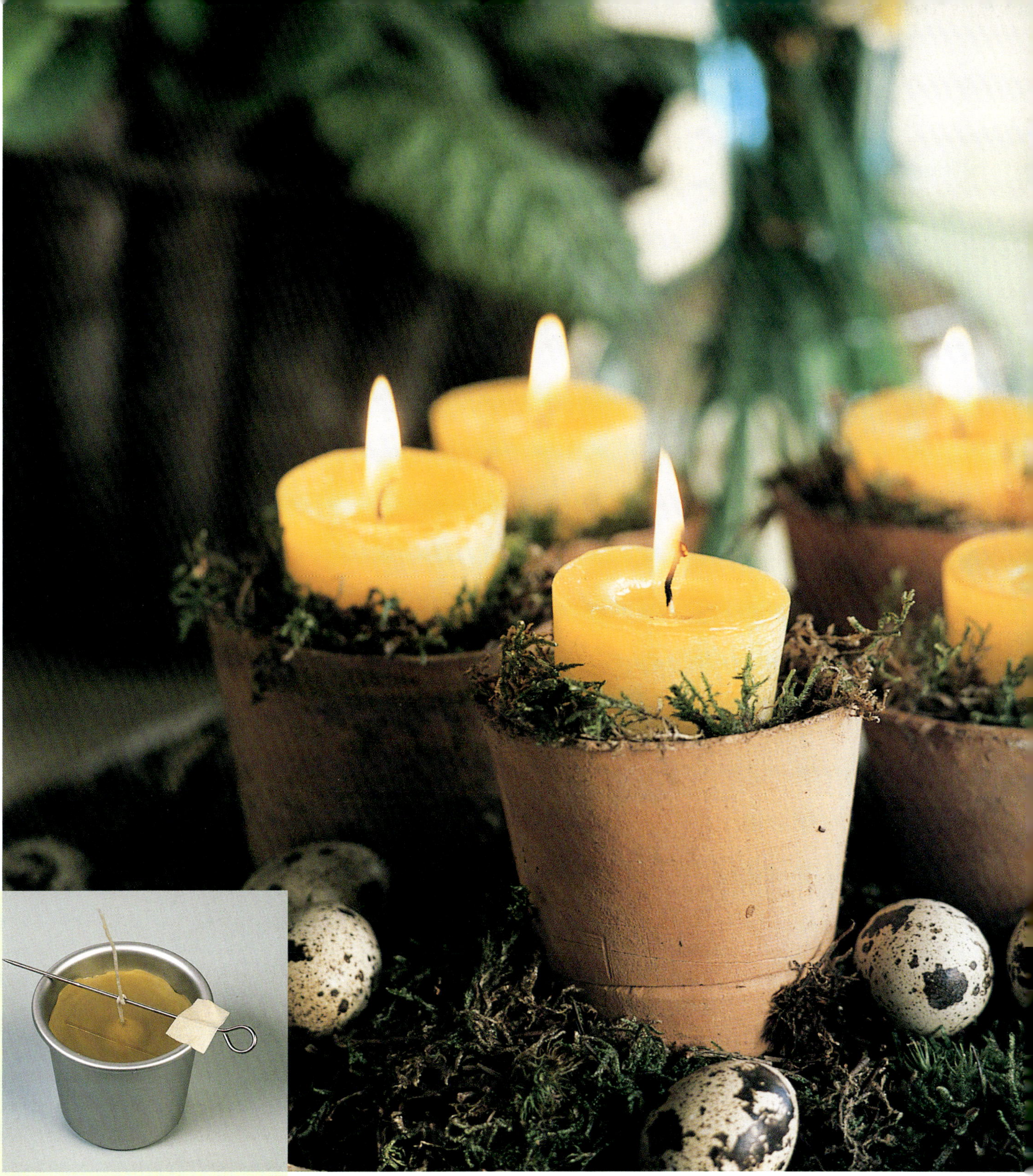

4 Fill the cavity that appears on the surface of the candle as it sets with more molten wax, taking care that wax doesn't run down between the candle sides and the mold. When set, remove the candle from the mold and trim the wick.

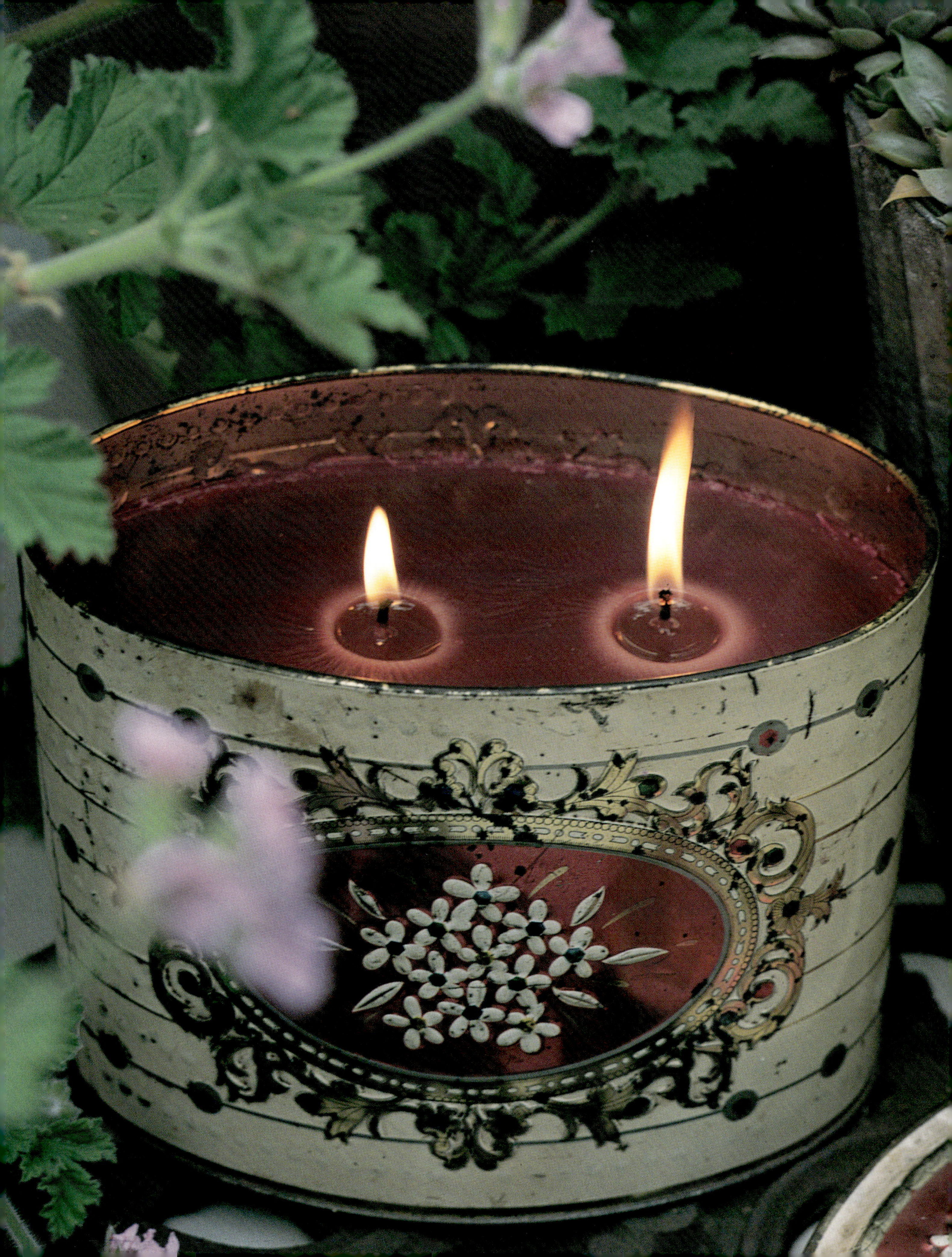

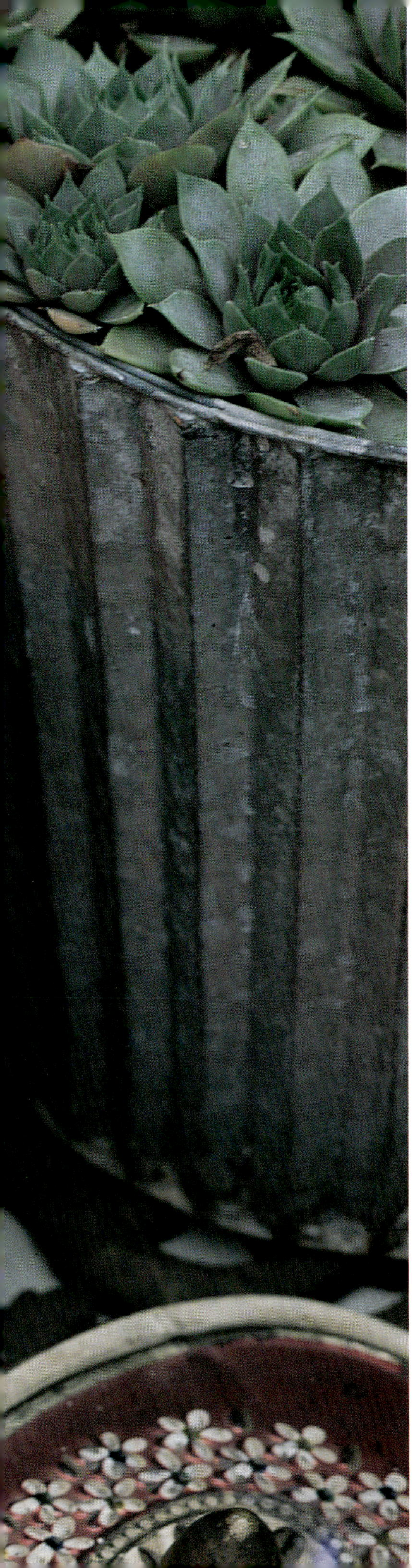

An oval tea tin is big enough for two wicks, bringing extra illumination to an evening in the garden.

outdoor tin candles

As the weather improves and daylight hours increase, use candles in the garden to illuminate an outdoor table at dusk or to highlight a display of potted plants. Recycle patterned Mediterranean olive oil cans or plain ridged tin cans as containers for stunning candles that can be left out in all weathers and will last throughout the season. Here, an inexpensive, old, patterned tea tin found in an antique store makes an ideal container and, when not in use, has a lid to keep the wicks dry when it rains. Add a combination of fresh herbal scents with a floral note to accentuate the natural scents that are just starting to make their presence felt in the warm evening air, such as peppermint and rosemary for their cooling and refreshing qualities and geranium to add balance and calm.

The metallic surface inside a tin reflects an extra glow from the light of the flame to great advantage as the candle burns and intensifies the illumination. For a party or leisurely evening eating in the garden, you need a candle that can burn for several hours—but do take care, as the surrounding metal will become very hot. Place candles where there is no danger of them being knocked over by passing adults or playful children, and put them only on surfaces that can take the heat from hot metal without causing any damage. If in doubt, protect surfaces with a perfectly flat ceramic tile or slab of marble placed underneath the candle. Even after the flame is extinguished, do not try to move the container until it has cooled sufficiently. When the candle has burned down, the container can be refilled in the same way as the original candle was made, again and again.

you will need:

Prepared medium container wick
2 wick sustainers
Tea tin or tin can
2½ lb. paraffin wax beads
Wax dye
Approximately 2½ fl. oz. essential oils or wax perfume

MAKING THE CANDLE Larger cans can take more than one wick, which gives extra illumination from glimmering flames. Use special container wicks so they can withstand the heat of the enclosed molten wax. The best way to extinguish the flame of container candles is by "drowning" the wick, as smoldering wicks sometimes burn right down to the surface of the candle and become unusable. Use a metal implement to push the lighted wick into the pool of wax that surrounds it to snuff it out cleanly, then return the wick to an upright position. The wick will then be primed and ready to light the next time. When recycling tin containers into candle holders, make sure they are clean and dry and any lids have been removed cleanly without leaving any jagged edges. Calculate the amount of wax you will need for your container as described on page 93. This tea tin measures 6 inches long by 3½ inches wide and 4½ inches high.

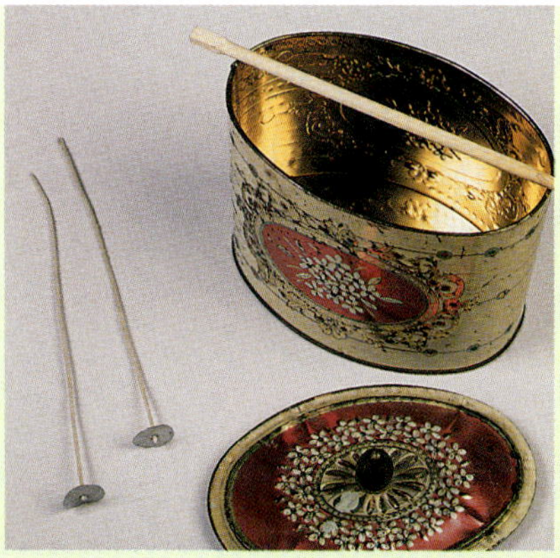

1 Cut two wicks to the depth of the container, allowing an extra inch on each. Thread one end of each wick through a wick sustainer and close the metal hole around the wick with pliers to secure. Trim the wicks flat to the base of each sustainer.

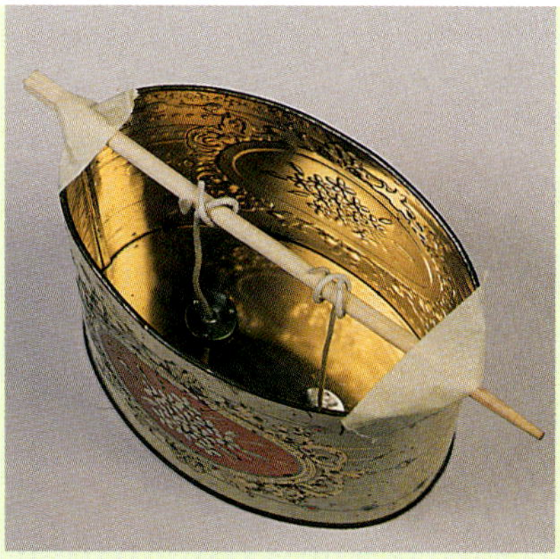

2 Position the wicks in the container so the sustainers sit on the bottom, winding the excess wick around a stick or wicking needle held steady across the top of the container with tape.

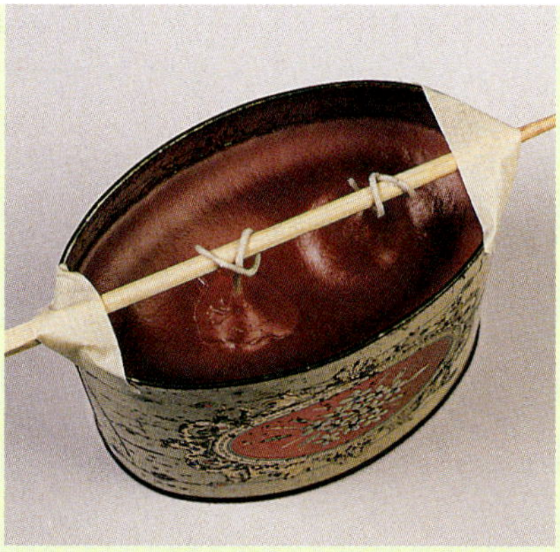

3 Melt the wax and dye together and heat to 180°F. Add the perfume and stir in. Pour the molten wax into the container, filling to within 1 inch of the rim. Allow to cool completely.

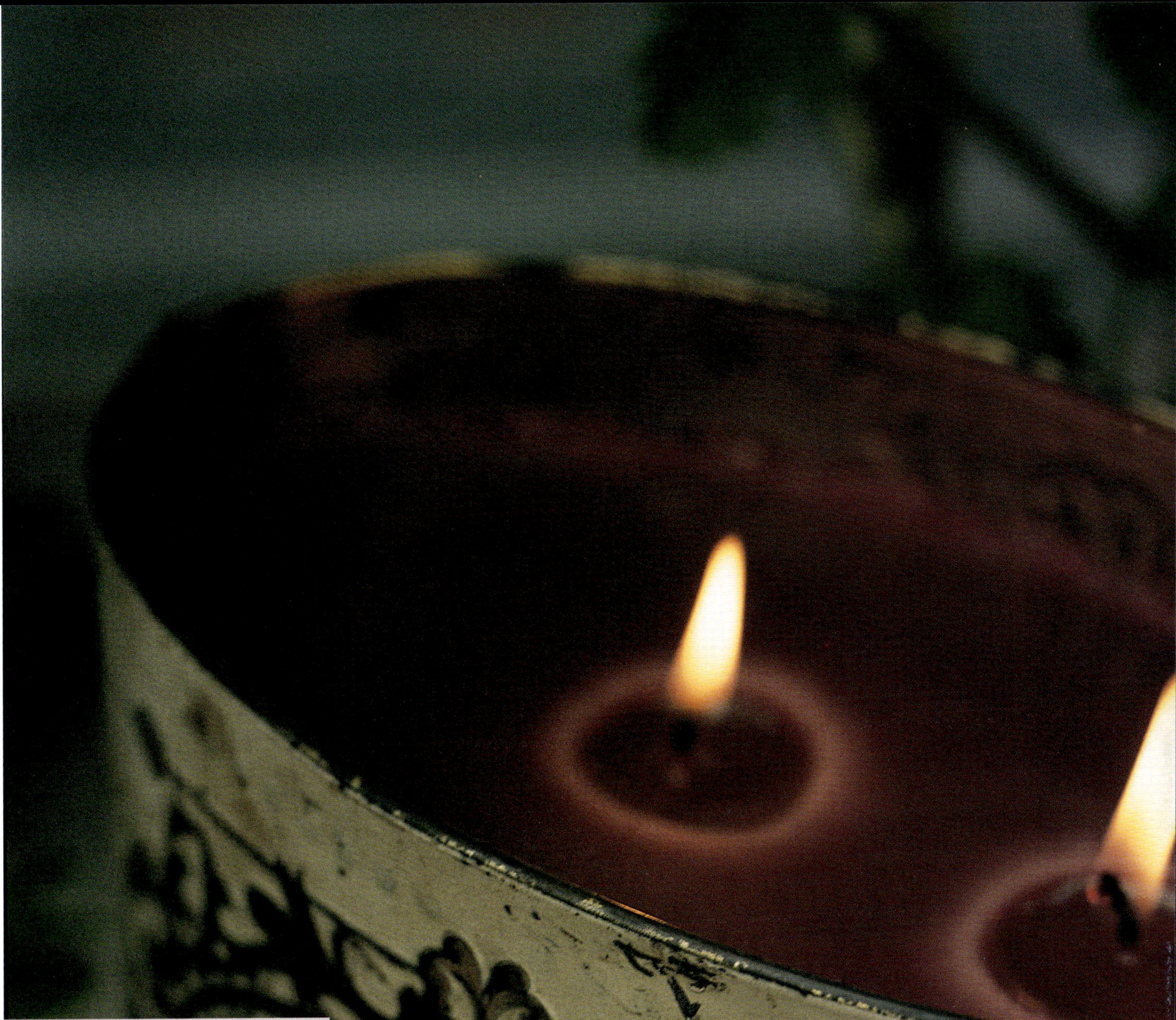

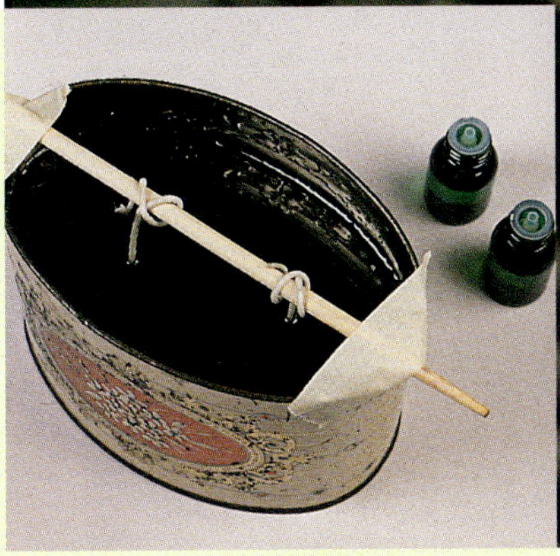

4 As the wax cools, it will shrink down around the wicks. Reheat the remaining wax to 180°F and pour the molten wax into the cavities. Allow to cool completely, then remove the stick and trim the wicks.

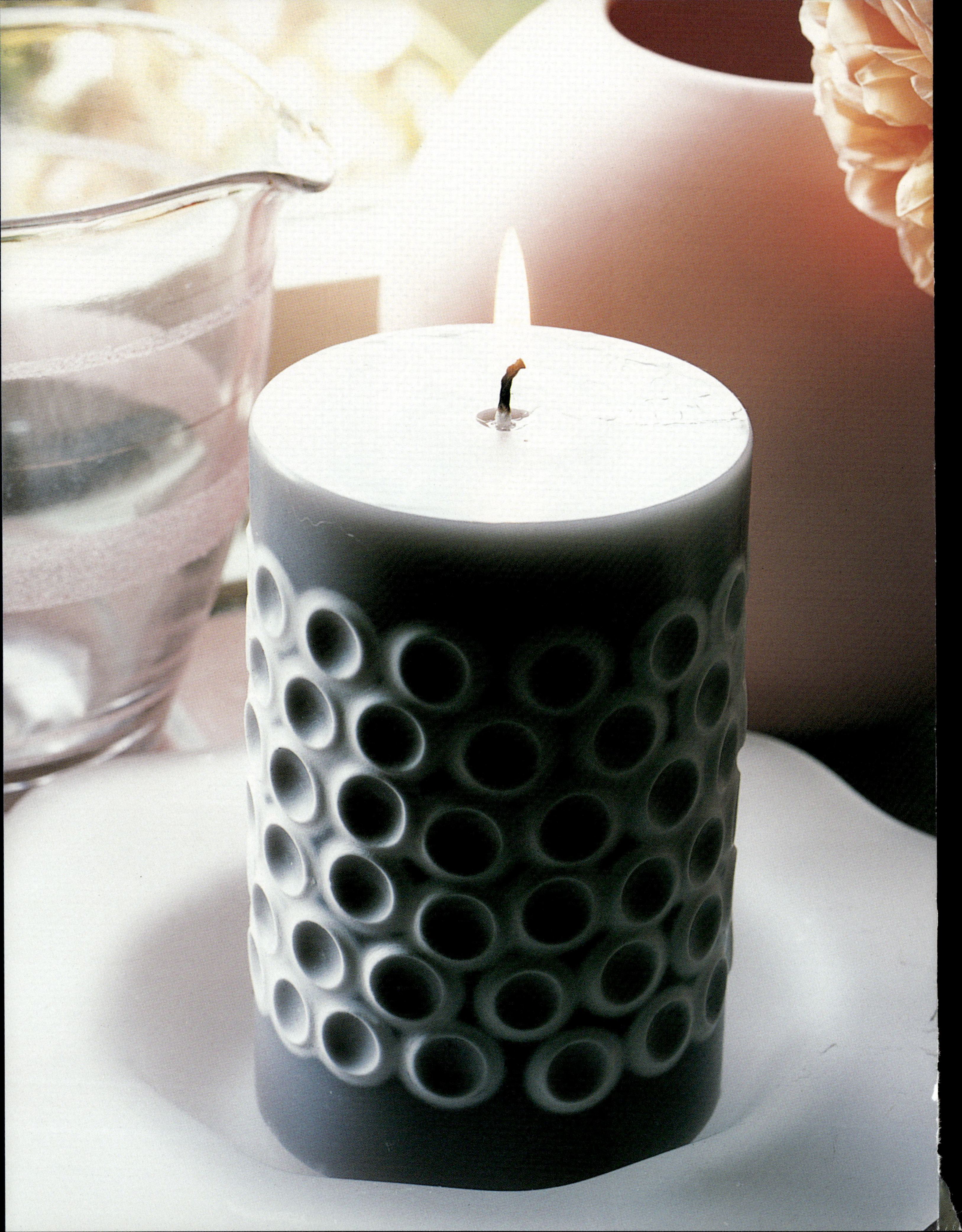

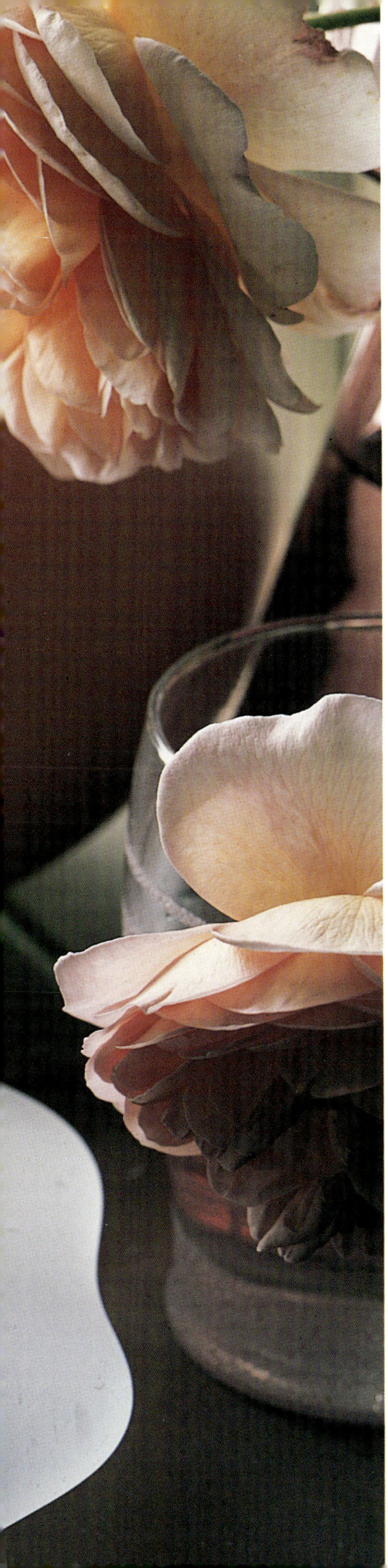

The craters on the wax surface, created with hammer blows applied to the cold candle, have an organic quality.

1960s candle

A hammer-beaten finish applied to a candle turns a simple pillar candle into a stylish and sculptural room accessory. The strong retro look of this candle captures the essence of the sixties. It would look good displayed alongside the similarly shaped vases and hand-blown glassware produced during that era, a style that has recently seen a revival and is exerting its influence upon fashionable home-furnishing design. The candle is scented with a modern combination of fragrances that are clean and leafy—a blend of cooling lime, calming geranium, and basil to restore and refresh.

The beaten texture on this candle has a tactile quality. The indentations are formed by the ball end of a hammer resting against the candle's surface being given a firm blow with a mallet. As the wax is displaced and pushed forward, it forms a pale, opaque circle, and the rows of circles resemble the tentacles of an octopus. Forming each crater one by one in alternating rows produces an unusual decorative band. The candle is scented with a combination of perfumes that are trendy and easy to live with.

you will need:

- Pillar candle mold
- Prepared wick
- Wicking needle
- 4½ oz. stearin
- Wax dye
- 1 lb. paraffin wax beads
- 1 fl. oz. essential oil or wax perfume
- Felt tip pen
- Ball-ended hammer
- Rubber mallet
- Ethyl alcohol
- Soft cloth

MAKING THE CANDLE Beating the indentations onto the candle needs to be done with a sure hand. Each mark requires only one determined strike from a rubber mallet against the hammer top. Try out the technique first on a spare candle, or keep the practice blows to a small area on the candle so the marks can be turned out of sight if they aren't successful. Don't try to repeat a blow in the same spot as this could cause the candle to crack. The textured effect is most successful on dark to midtone colors as the displaced wax forms a pale rim around each crater, which shows up best against a stronger, contrasting shade. This mold measures 3¼ inches in diameter and 5 inches in height.

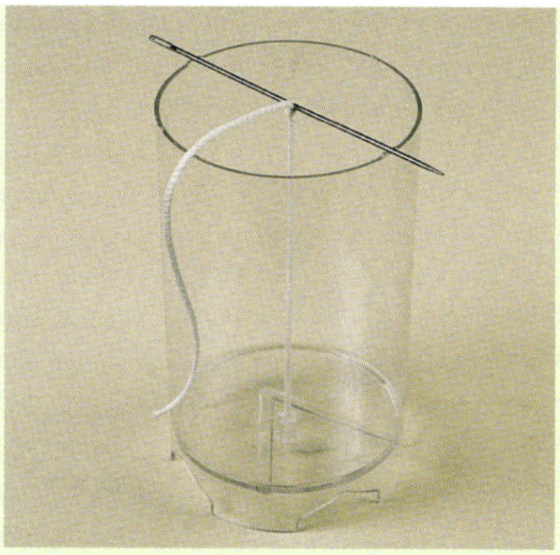

1 Prepare the mold by threading the wick through the base, then knot the wick in place. Seal to make it watertight. Place the wicking needle across the top of the mold and tie the wick on tightly to hold it in place.

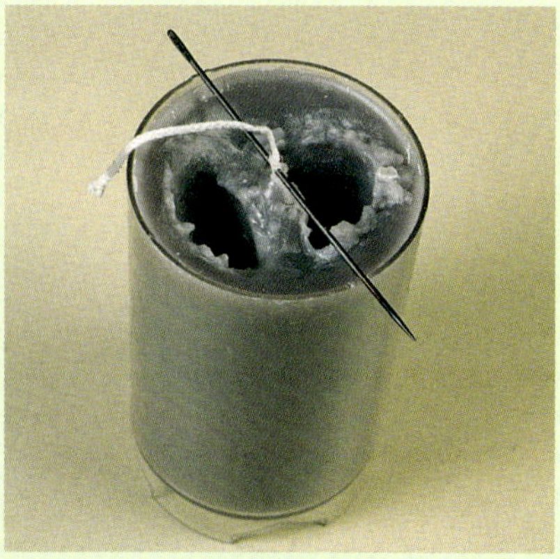

3 When the wax has set, cavities will appear around the wick. Reheat the wax as before and fill the cavities, making sure that wax doesn't run over the edges between the candle and the mold. Allow to cool completely.

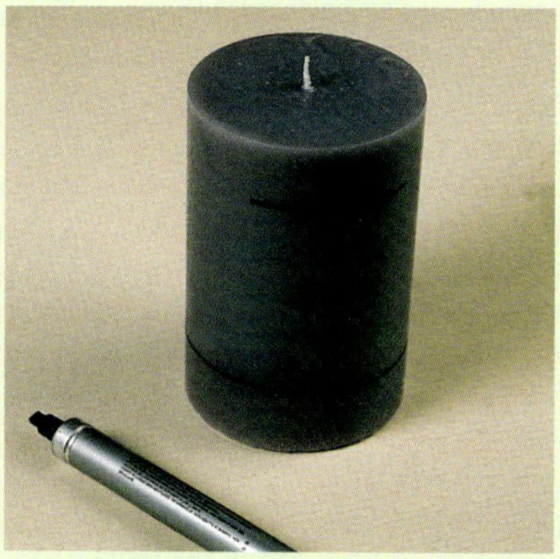

4 Remove the candle from the mold and trim the wick. If necessary, smooth the top with a hot iron to remove any marks in the wax. After you have finished with the iron, run it along newspaper while it is still warm to clean it and remove any excess wax. Draw two horizontal lines around the candle with a felt tip pen to mark the outer edges of the decorative band.

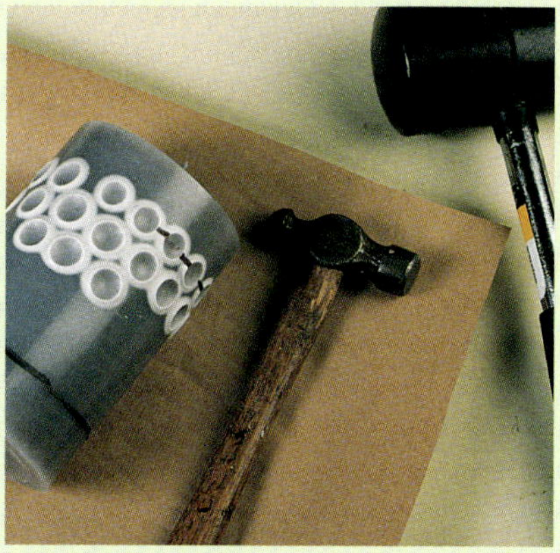

5 Using the top line as a guide, place the ball end of the hammer centrally on the line and strike the other end of the hammer top once firmly with the rubber mallet to form a crater. Repeat to make more craters in rows.

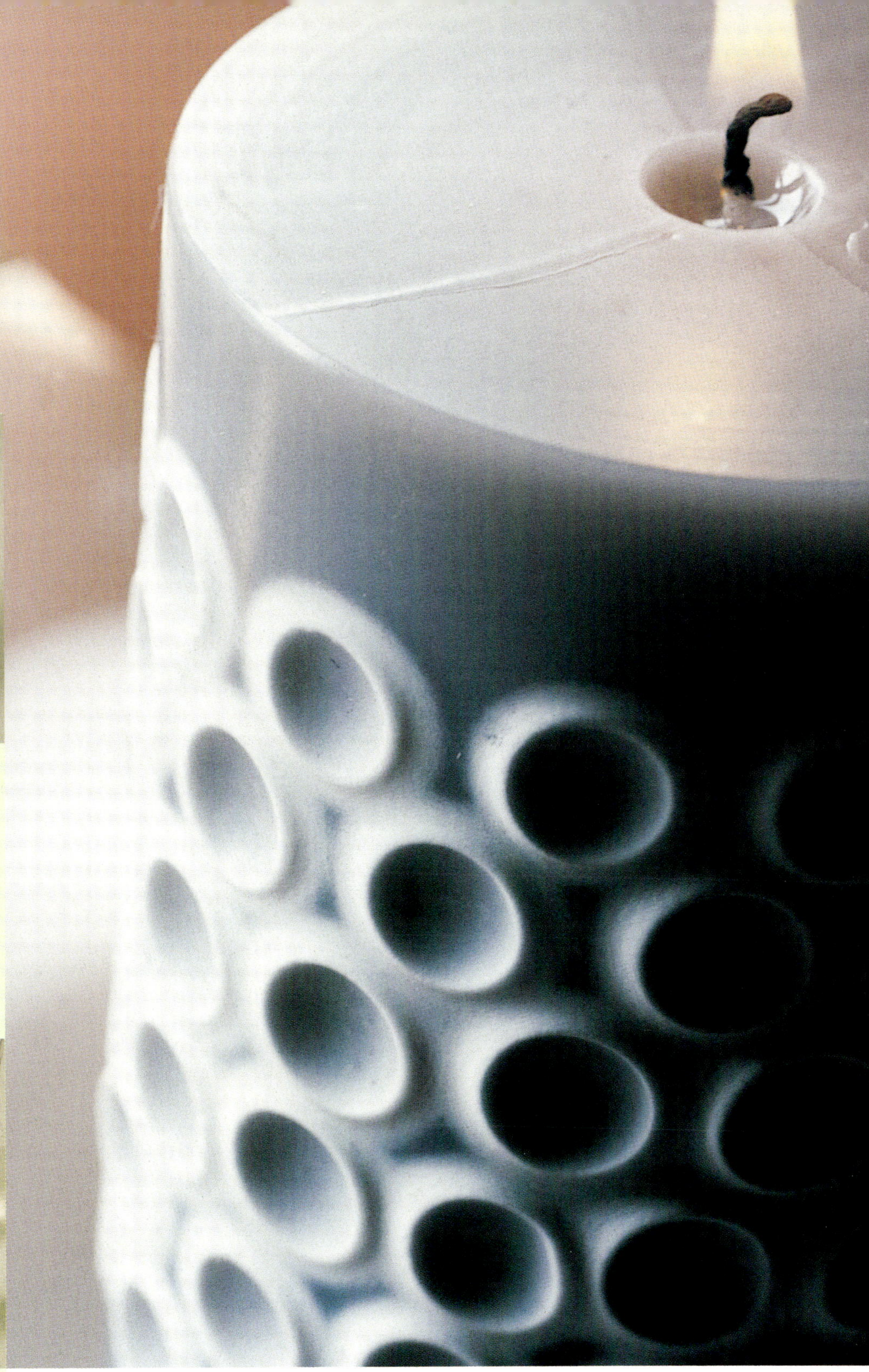

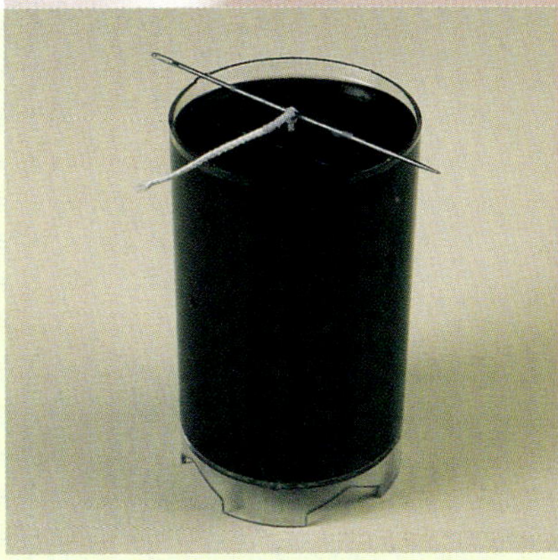

2 Melt the stearin with the dye in the top of a double boiler and add the wax. Heat to to 200°F. Add the perfume and mix in. Pour the molten wax into the mold, then cool in a water bath.

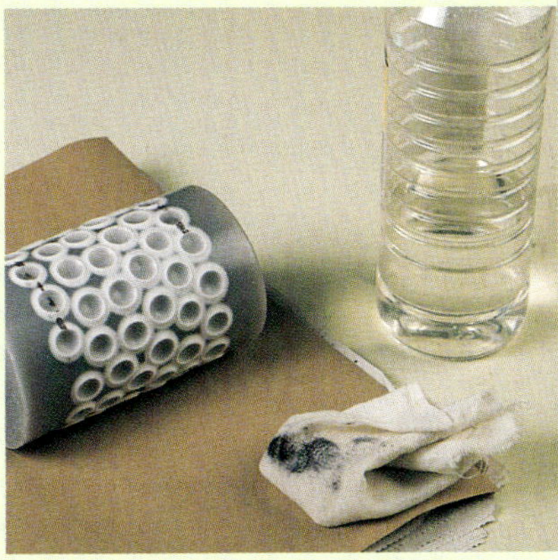

6 When the central decorative band is completely filled with rows of craters, clean away the felt tip pen lines using a soft cloth and ethyl alcohol.

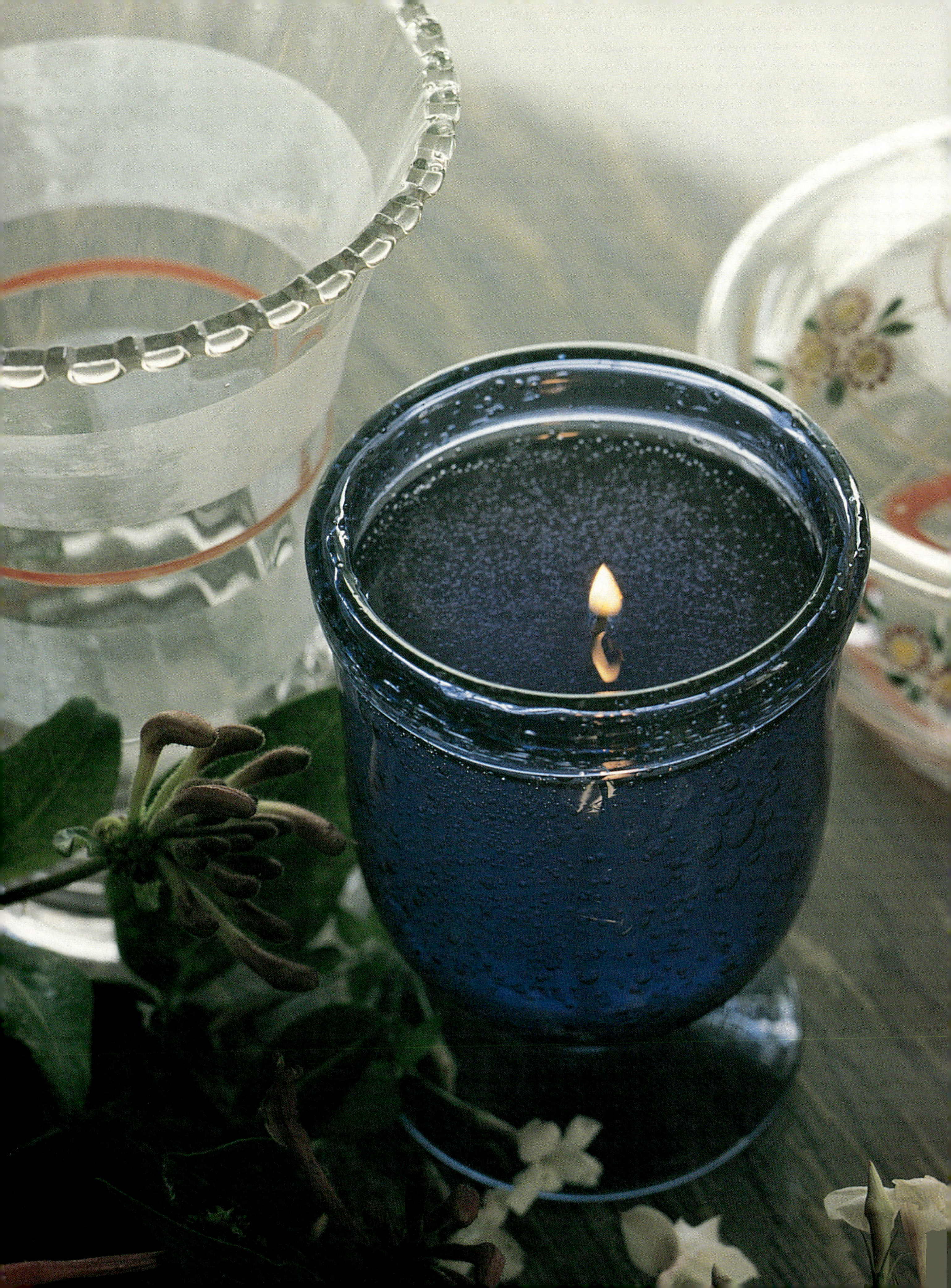

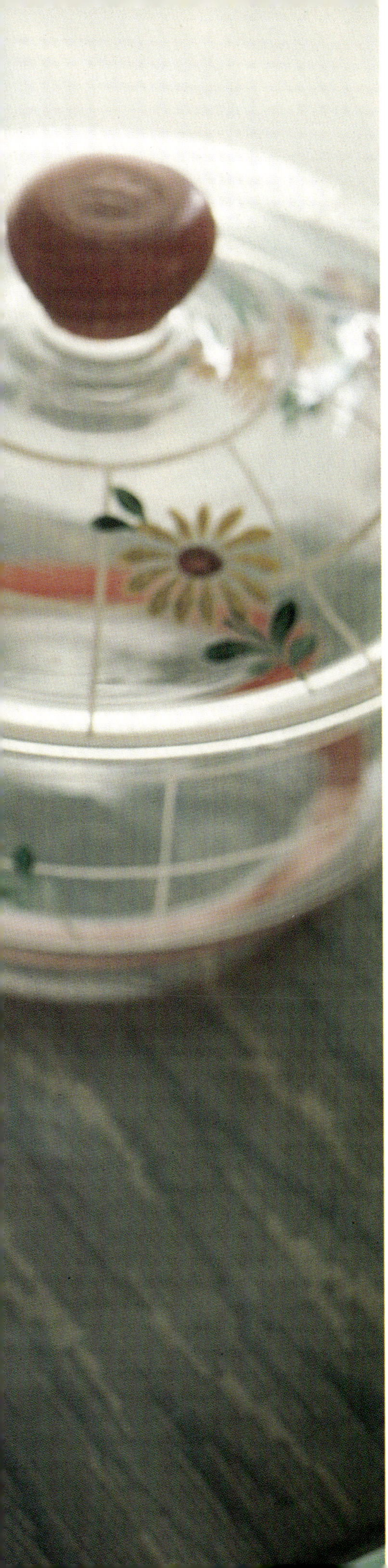

Use colored glass tumblers to make pretty containers for gel candles that make an attractive display alongside other glass vases and dishes.

gel container candle

Using gel to make candles must surely be the simplest technique from the candlemaker's repertoire. The transparency and delicacy of this material make it ideal for filling glass containers, and the light from the flame will shine through the translucent colors of the glassware. The gel candle shown here uses a hand-blown goblet; the bubbles sealed within the glass surface accentuate the bubbling quality of the gel, which has been dyed a deep shade of purple to complement the container. The lightness of these materials perfectly suits the delicate floral scents of honeysuckle and jasmine, a soothing and romantic combination.

Make your candle using colored gel to add vibrancy to a simple clear-glass container. Alternatively, fill a tinted drinking glass with clear gel so the colors glow through. Candle gel is easy to handle and pulls away from surfaces cleanly when it has set. Bubbles usually form in the molten gel—while some people view this as a desired quality, others see it as a problem. Gel is now available in different grades, including "bubble-free," which is preferred. This gel still needs to be handled gently or some bubbles will still form. It can also be bought already colored, which removes the degree of guesswork, but it is also easy to dye it using wax pigment to add the color. Unlike with paraffin wax, where the molten color usually looks completely different when it's cold, with gel the color looks the same shade whether liquid or set. Whatever glass container you choose, it must be able to withstand the heat of melted gel.

you will need:

- Prepared wick
- Wick sustainer
- Glass container
- 7 oz. gel
- Small amount of pigment or wax dye
- 1 tsp. essential oil or candle perfume

MAKING THE CANDLE Use wax pigment to color the gel rather than wax dye, which makes gel look cloudy. Pure pigment is available in granules, and just a sprinkle added to the molten gel can produce a good coloration, so always add the pigment with a light hand. If you are intending to make just one or two candles and can only buy the pigment in large quantities, it will be more economical to buy your gel pre-colored. When making lots of gel candles, prepare batches of strongly pigmented gel and store it in sealed plastic containers. When you need to color a candle, simply break off a small piece of the pigmented gel and add it to molten clear gel. To work out how much gel you will need, roughly pack your container with broken-up gel, then add a little extra. Clean the container afterward with soapy water so it sparkles before making the candle. This glass container measures 2¾ inches in diameter and 3¼ inches high.

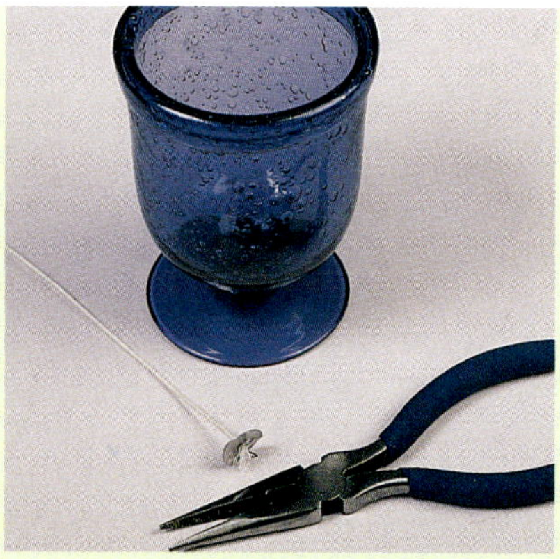

1 Cut the wick to the depth of the glass plus a bit extra. Attach the wick sustainer to one end of the wick, using long pliers to close the sustainer and fix it firmly in place.

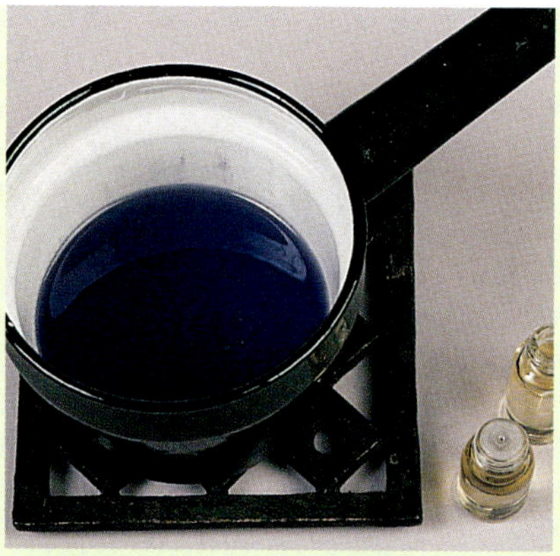

2 Put enough gel to fill your container into the pan and warm gently over a low heat until it melts. Add the wax pigment little by little until the required color is achieved. Heat the molten gel to 220°F and add the perfume.

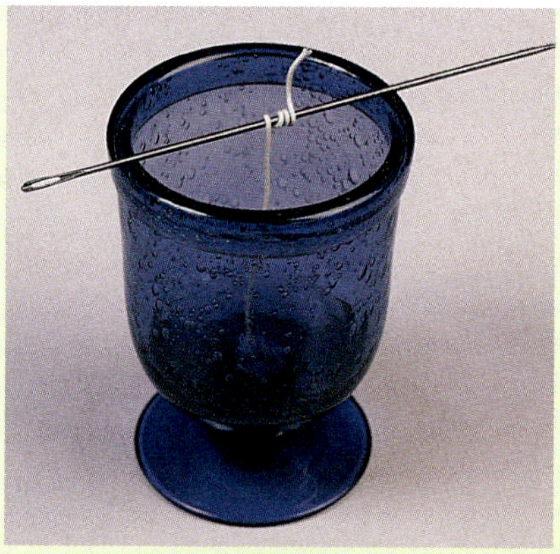

3 Place the wick centrally in the container so the sustainer sits on the bottom and wrap the excess wick around a wicking needle sitting across the rim of the glass.

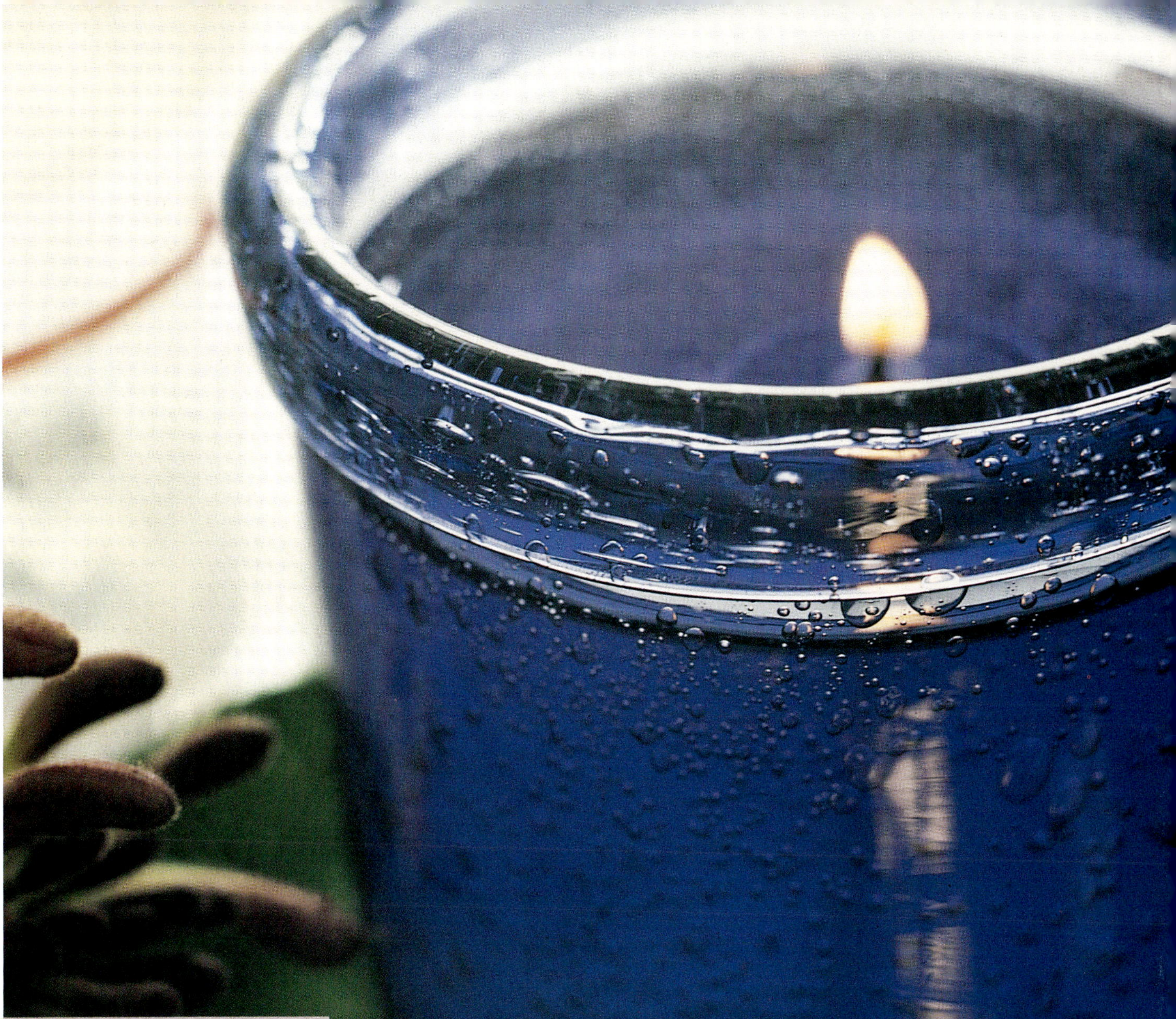

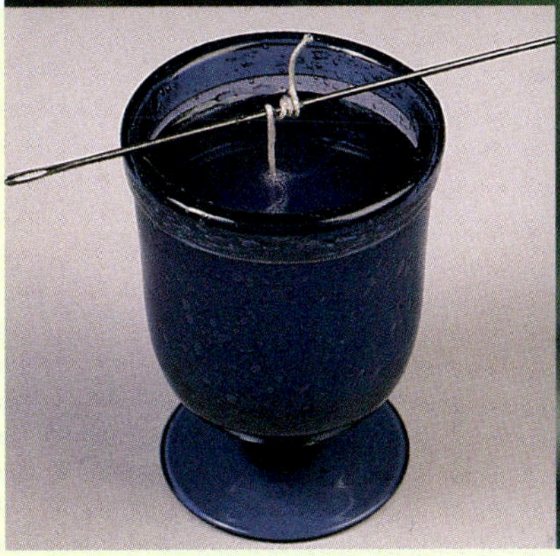

4 Pour the gel into the container, taking care to avoid splashing the sides to give a good clean edge. Allow to completely set. Remove the wicking needle and trim the wick.

From the softest, palest pink of early spring to the deeper, warmer shades of the later months, pink is the color seen in nature as spring gradually turns to summer, and the garden truly comes to life.

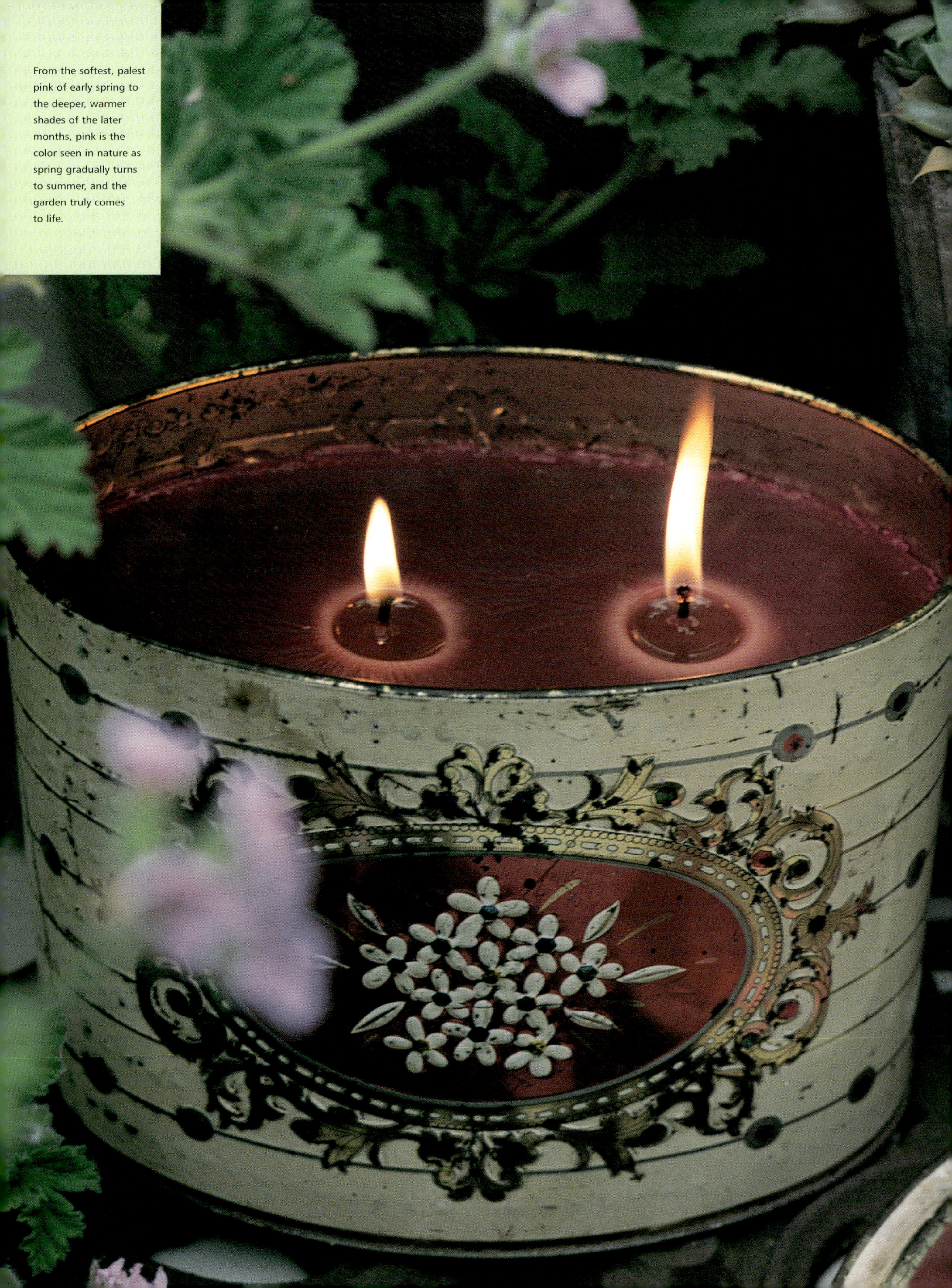

SPRING COLORS

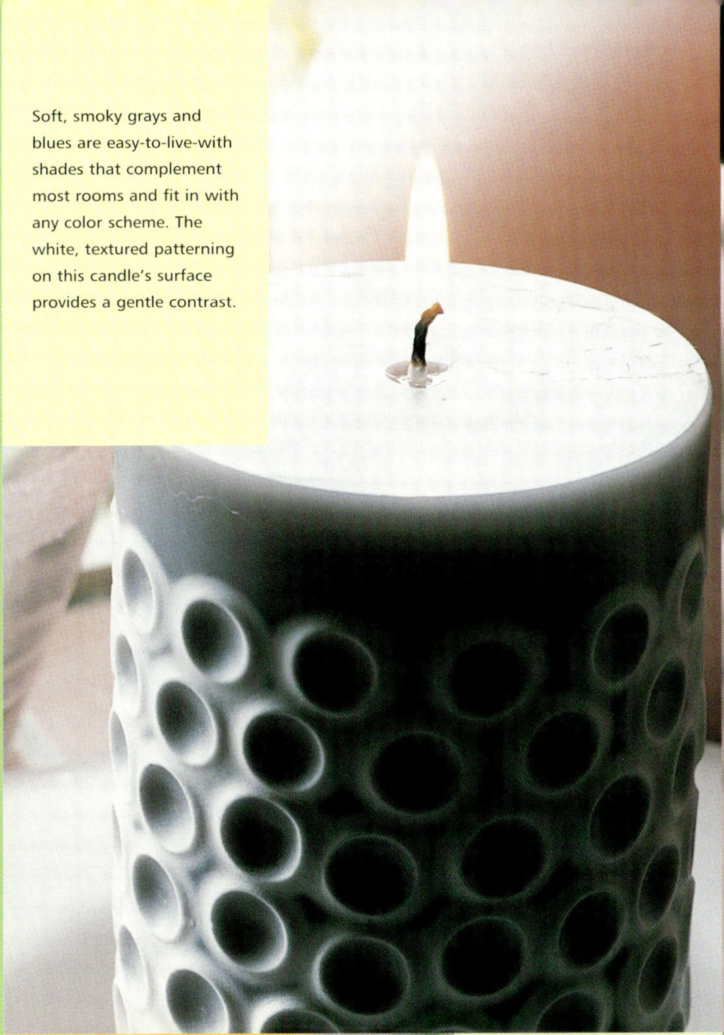

Soft, smoky grays and blues are easy-to-live-with shades that complement most rooms and fit in with any color scheme. The white, textured patterning on this candle's surface provides a gentle contrast.

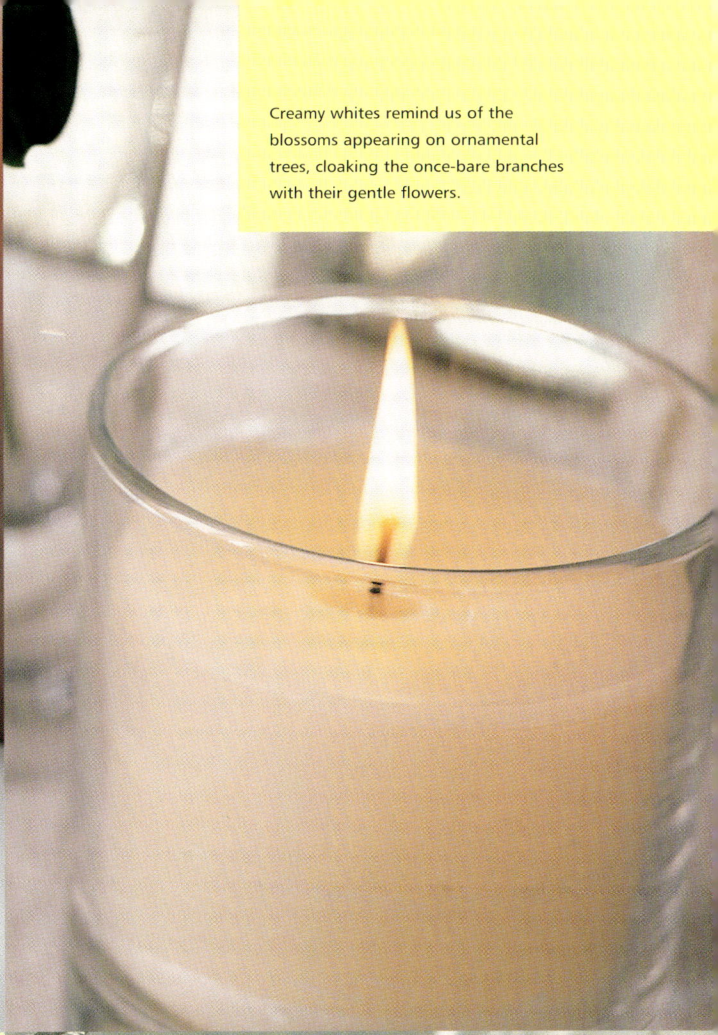

Creamy whites remind us of the blossoms appearing on ornamental trees, cloaking the once-bare branches with their gentle flowers.

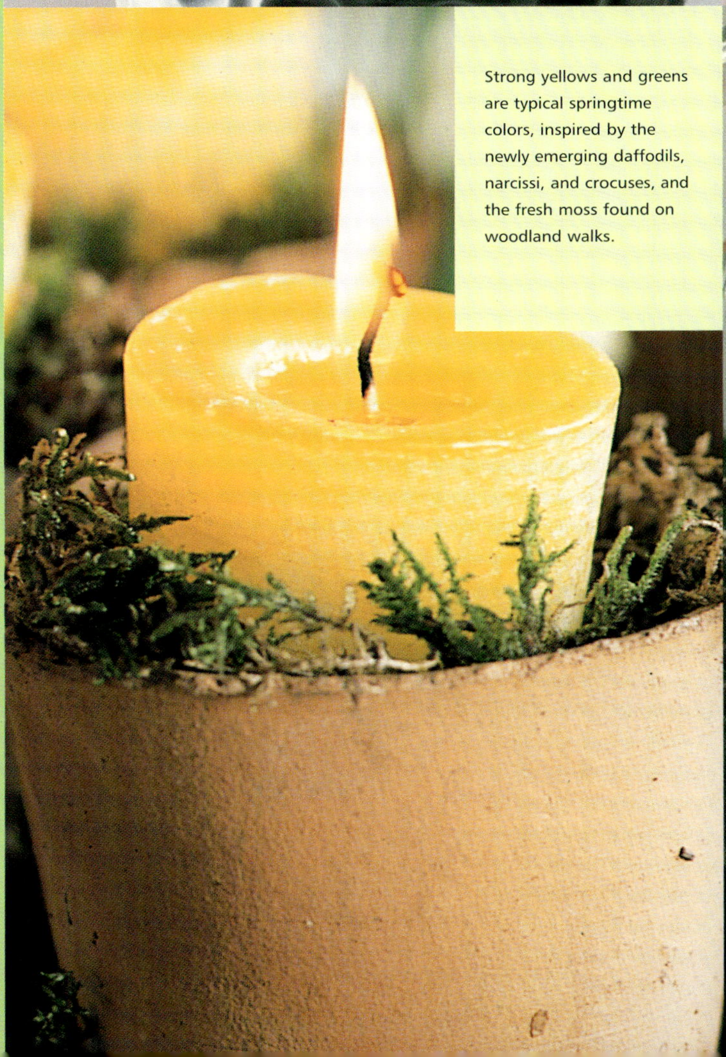

Strong yellows and greens are typical springtime colors, inspired by the newly emerging daffodils, narcissi, and crocuses, and the fresh moss found on woodland walks.

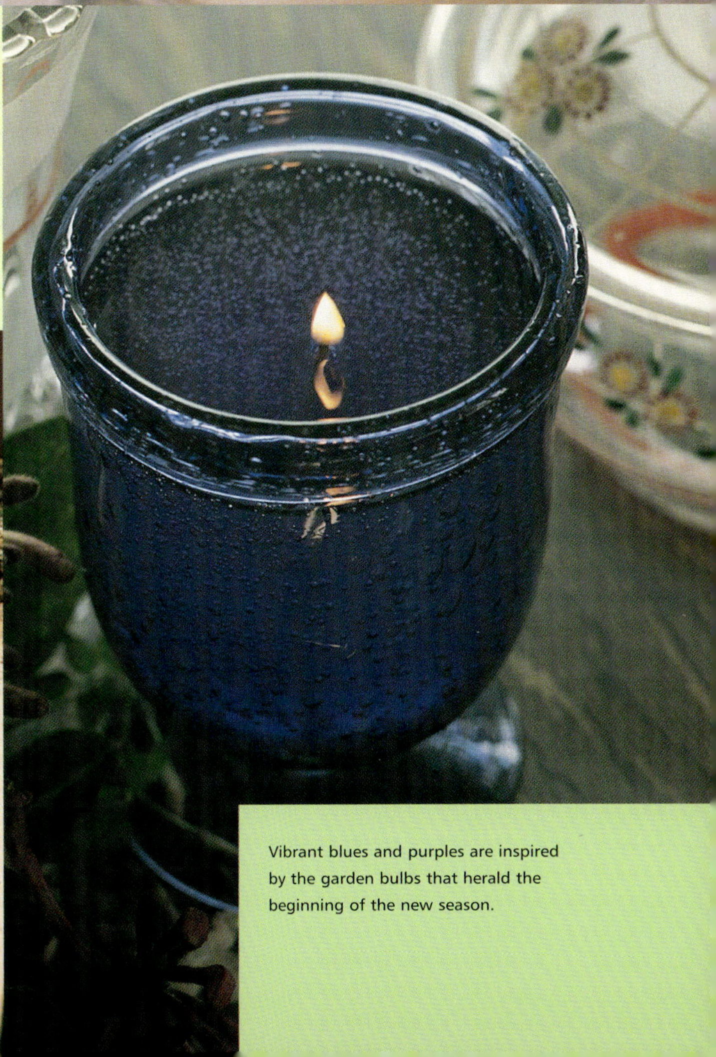

Vibrant blues and purples are inspired by the garden bulbs that herald the beginning of the new season.

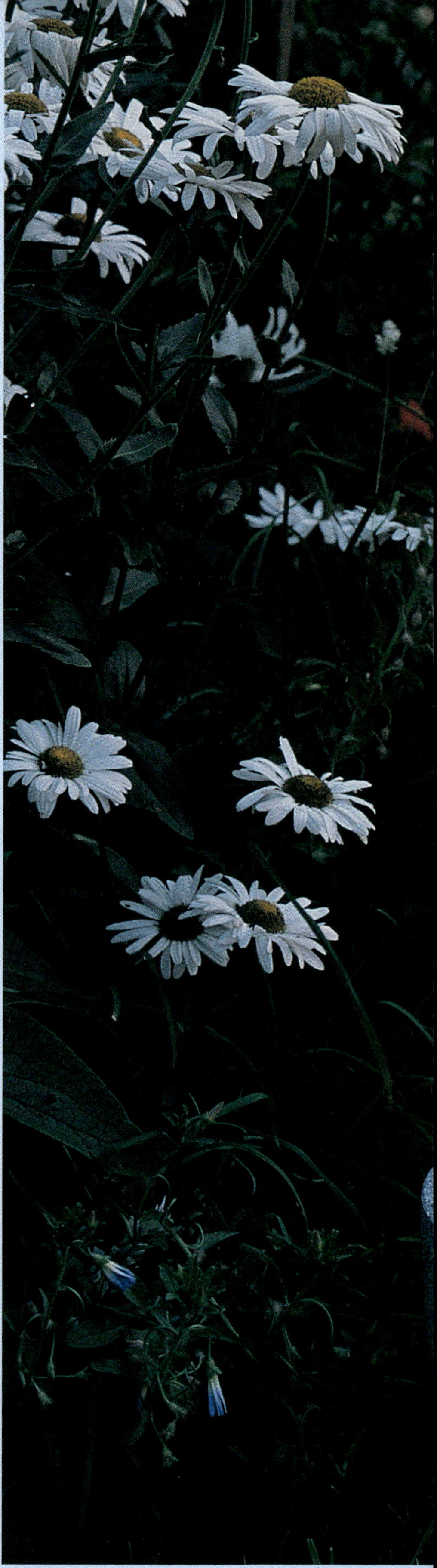

ESSENCE OF summer

By day the leaves of plants and herbs are warmed by the sun, by dusk the medley of fragrances from the garden begins to make its delicious impact. Now the garden bursts into bloom with a riot of colors and scents. Old garden roses unfurl beautiful, crumpled petals, their light, powdery aroma filling the air with fragrant notes of sherbet, vanilla, and musk. The delicate aromas of jasmine, honeysuckle, sweet peas, and tobacco plants carry on the breeze on balmy evenings. Later in the season, spires of lavender rise above the herbaceous border, their flowers filled with richly scented oil. Now is the time to mirror these marvelous qualities of the season in the home.

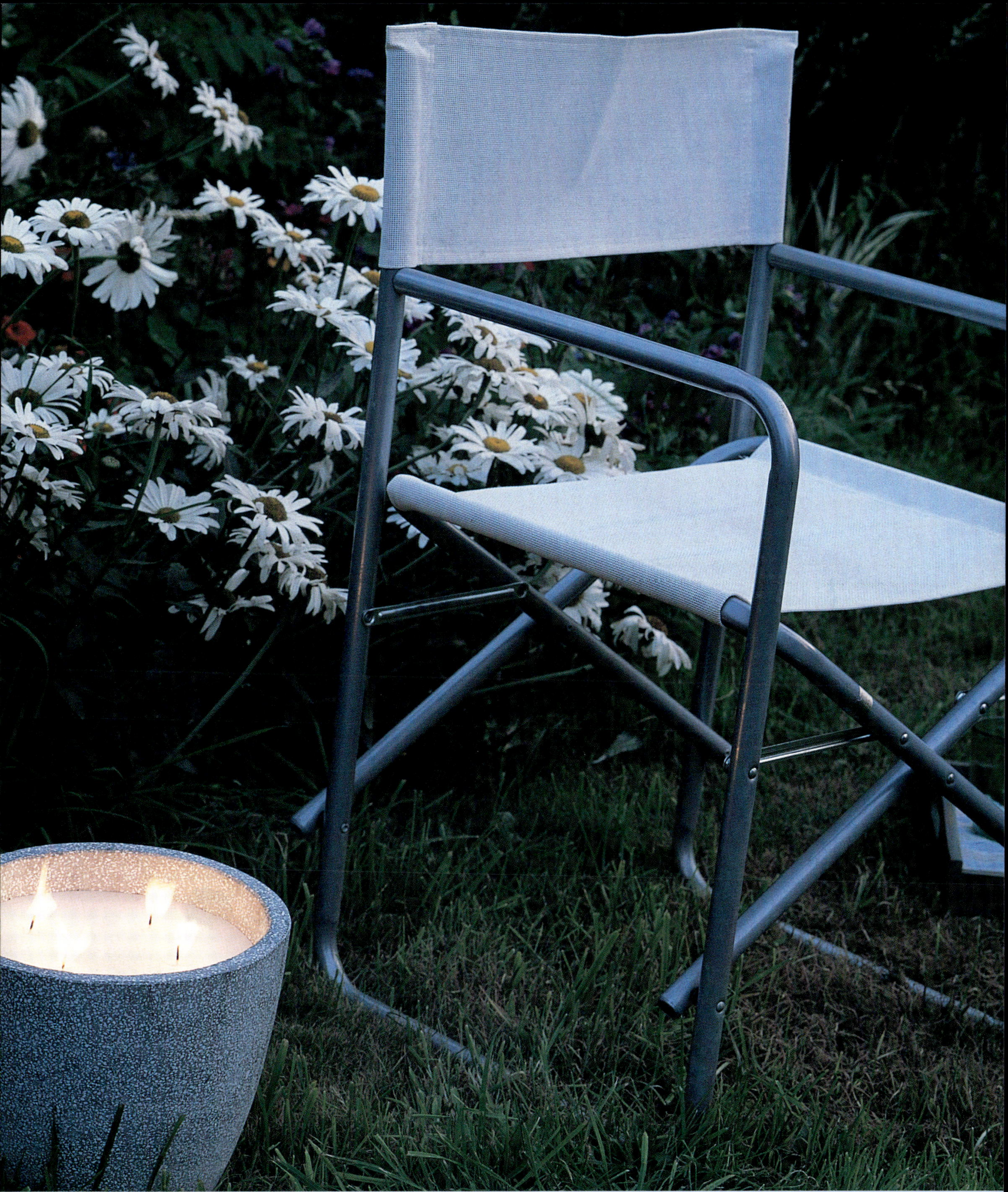

A comfortable chair set in a favorite place in the garden, where the delicate scent of flowers in full bloom mingles with the spicy perfume wafting from the candle.

Straight-sided candles are the classic choice for candlesticks and candelabras. They are surprisingly quick and easy to make as they set quickly. The big advantage of making your own is that you can tailor the colors to match your room or table linen, and the scents can be customized. Perfume individual candelabra candles with single scents so they can be burned together, creating your own fragrant blend. To choose combinations of scents, clutch several open bottles of oil together in one hand and waft them under your nose so the various notes mingle together. The subtle colors used here complement the delicate scents of vanilla, tuberose, and angelica.

candlestick candle

you will need:

- Prepared 1-inch wick
- Mold seal
- Glass candlestick candle mold
- ½ oz. stearin
- Wax dye
- 3½ oz. paraffin wax beads
- Approximately 1 tsp. essential oil or wax perfume

MAKING THE CANDLE The mold needs to be held steady as the wax is poured in and left to set, so a cardboard collar that holds the mold and rests on a stand is necessary. Make a collar by cutting a circle the same size as the diameter of the mold in a square of strong cardboard so the lip of the mold can't fall through. If you intend to make many candles, use plastic board or coat the cardboard with varnish to make it water resistant, so splashes from the water bath will not ruin it. Craft stores sell special tripods and stands to suspend candle molds, but a tall, straight vase would serve the same purpose. This mold measures ¾ inch in diameter and 8 inches in length.

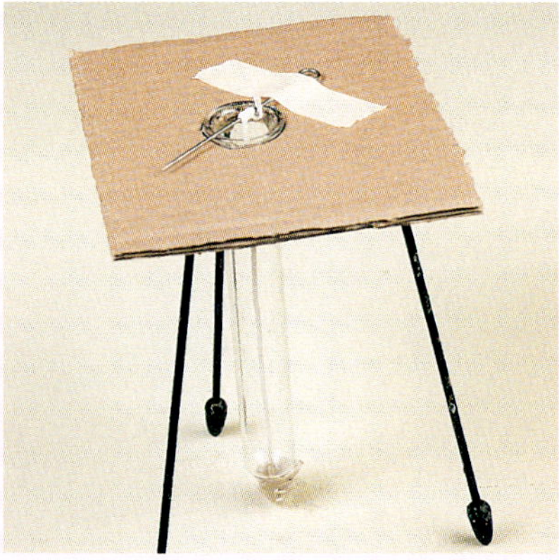

1 Thread the wick through the mold and securely seal the end with mold seal where it emerges. Tie the other end to a wicking needle to hold the wick tightly inside the mold. Make a collar out of cardboard to hold the mold in place and rest this across a tripod or stand.

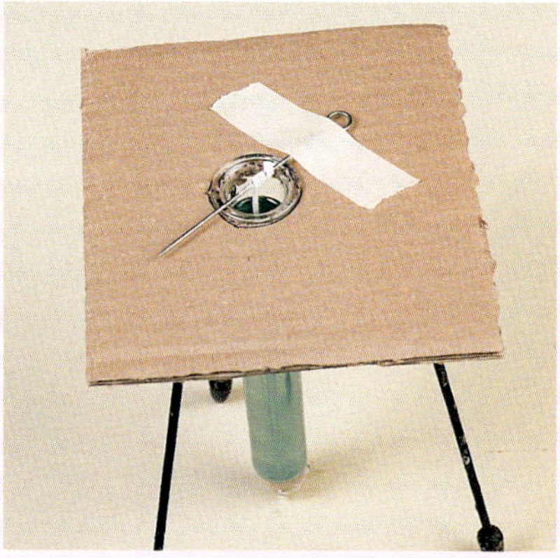

2 Melt the stearin in a double boiler and add the dye. When melted and combined, add the paraffin wax and heat the molten mixture to 200°F. Carefully pour the wax into the mold, right to the top.

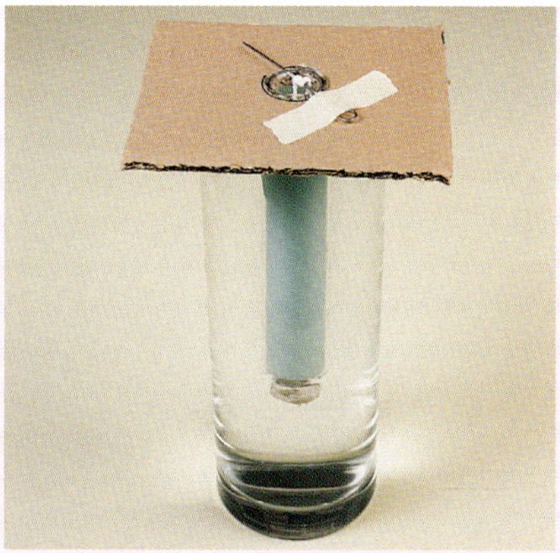

3 To cool the wax quickly so the surface is smooth and clear, use a vase deeper than the mold to make a water bath. Fill the vase with water and place the mold inside it so the collar rests across the vase's rim. Allow to set.

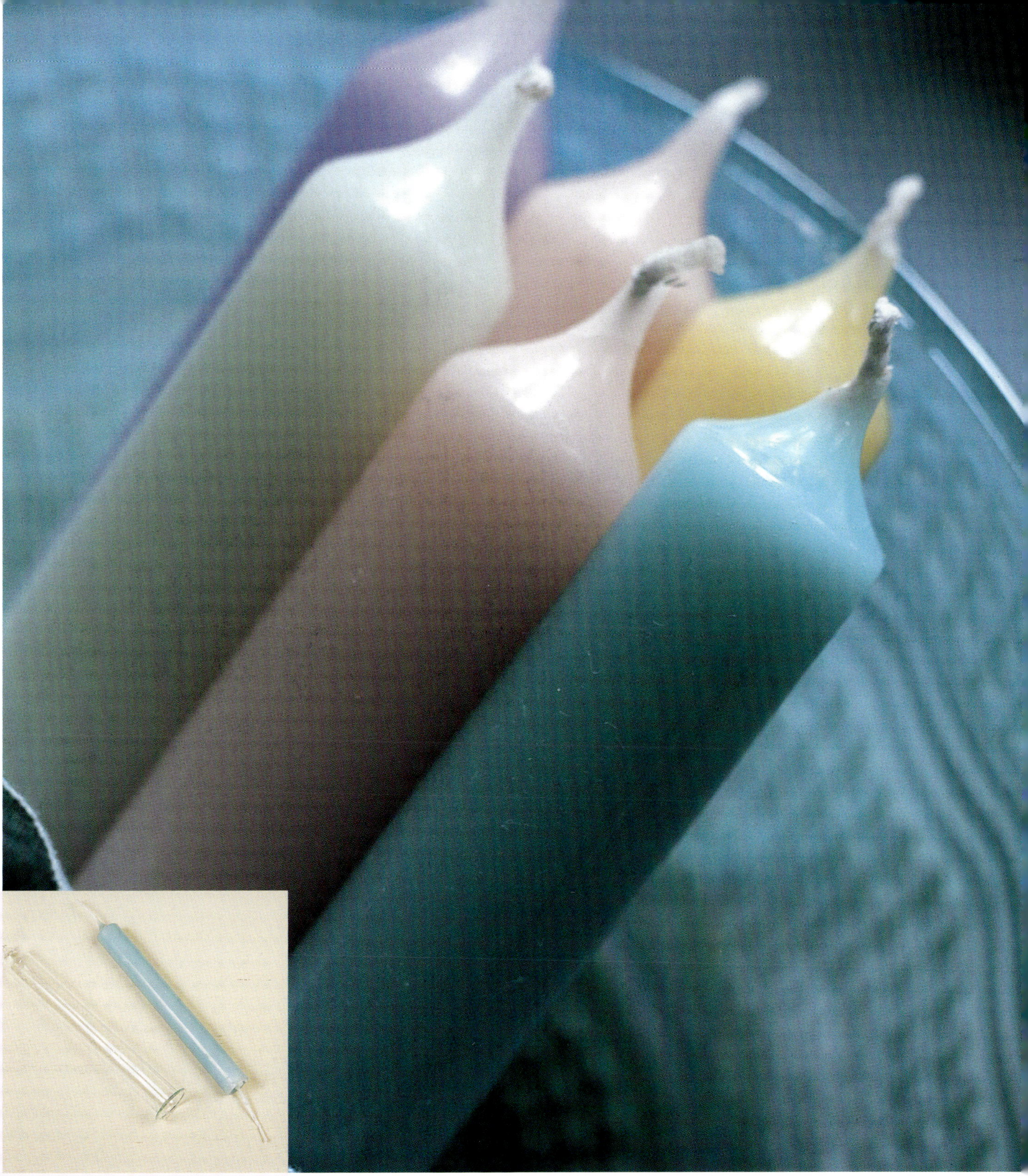

4 Reheat the wax and fill the dip around the wick. Allow to set, then remove the candle from the mold. Remove any mold seal left on the wick and trim it to ¾ inch. Smooth the base of the candle with a hot iron.

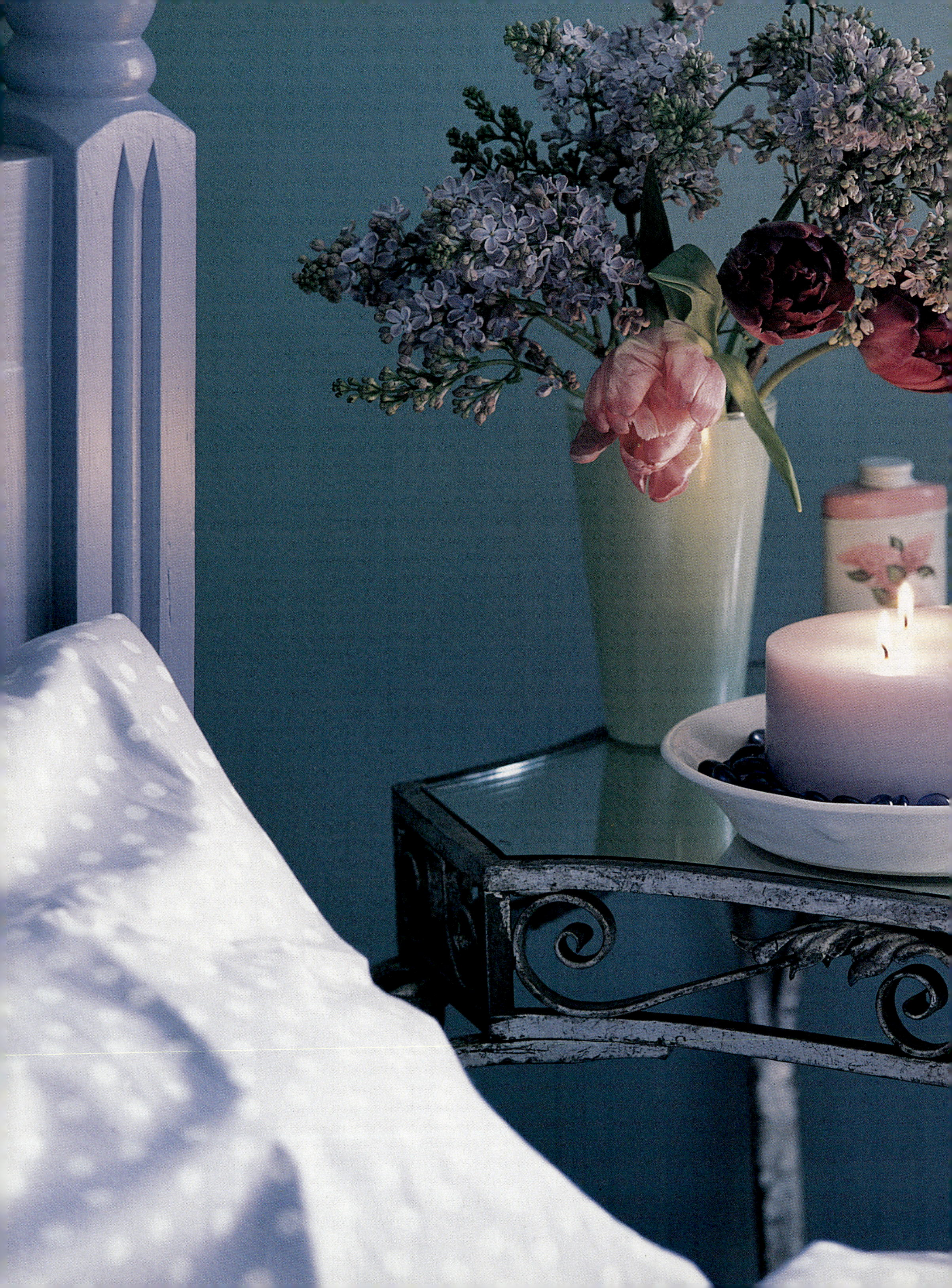

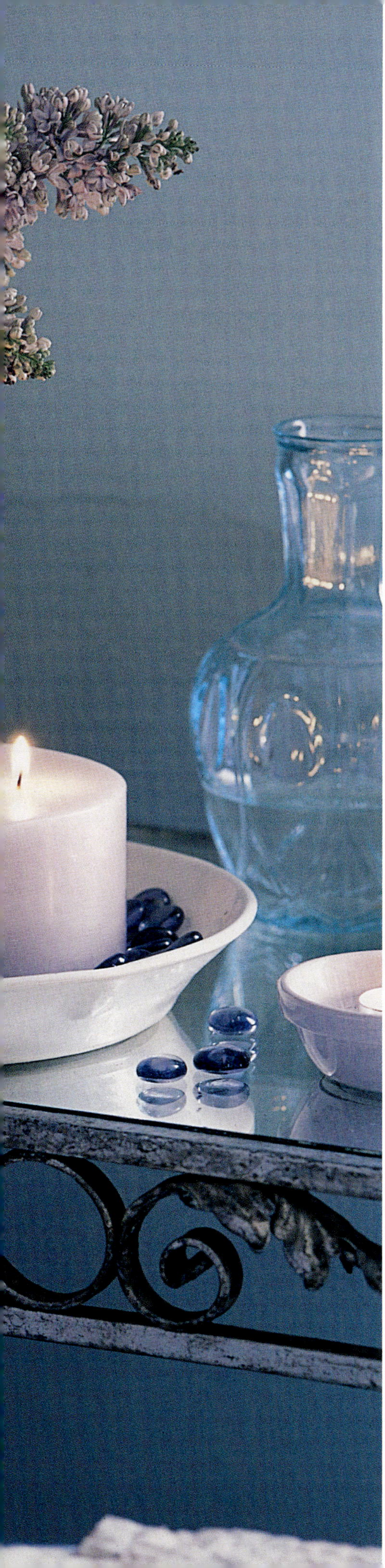

Wide candles can accommodate more than one wick, as there is enough room for several aromatic pools of wax to form.

multiwick candle

Bedrooms need to be comfort zones where we allow ourselves to heal and recharge. By choosing oils that are sleep-enhancing and rejuvenating, you will transform your room into a haven that feeds the mind and the body. Every part of a lavender plant is scented, and the oil distilled from the flower heads is particularly renowned for its relaxing and calming qualities. This fresh scent teams up readily with other perfumes: rose geranium makes a sensual, aromatic companion and complements the balancing and soothing characteristics. Make sure that any candles you use in a bedroom have a steady base and are placed in dishes, not directly on furniture, and most important, be sure to extinguish the flames before you fall blissfully asleep.

Large multiwicked candles have become fashionable home accessories but can be expensive to buy. One large, bold candle can look especially stylish and makes a definite statement when displayed in a bedroom or living room. It is always satisfying to be able to make something yourself that is just as good, if not better, than the store-bought version, and when you make your own you can customize the color and scents. Finding a mold suitable to make such a large, round candle can be a problem, as craft stores usually sell molds for smaller, standard designs. To find unusual molds, you simply need to be resourceful and see the potential in other containers that will do the job just as well, in this instance a paint bucket from a hardware store.

you will need:

Prepared medium wick
Suitable mold
Mold seal
7 oz. stearin
Wax dye
2¼ lb. paraffin wax beads
Approximately 2½ fl. oz. essential oils or wax perfume

MAKING THE CANDLE A paint bucket made of plastic or tin makes an ideal mold for this wide column candle. Look out for a container that is perfectly smooth inside, as any marks or ridges will be copied exactly on the surface of the wax. This candle is constructed so the bottom of the mold will be the top of the candle, so pay particular attention to the smoothness of the base and how sharp or rounded the inside corners are. Drill holes in the base of the mold using an electric or hand drill, making them just big enough to thread the wicks through—any bigger and it will be more difficult to make it watertight with mold seal, meaning the molten wax will seep out. The mold needs to be supported above the tabletop—a few wooden blocks will do the job perfectly well. After making the candle and removing it from the mold, use a hot iron to smooth the base. Make sure you remove any mold seal from around the wicks or it will be difficult to light them. This mold measures 6¼ inches in diameter with a depth of 4¾ inches.

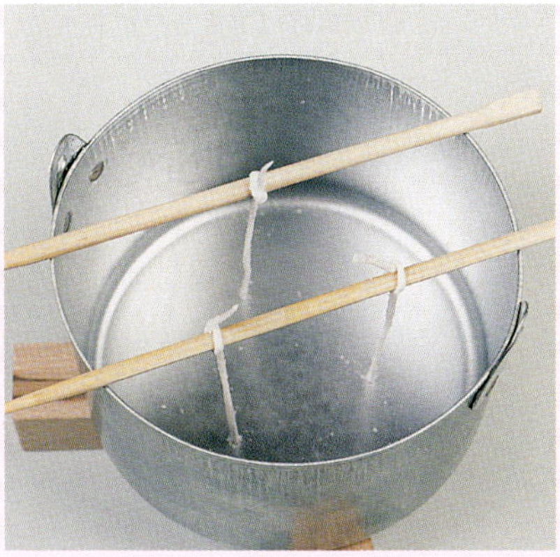

1 Thread the wicks through the holes in the base of the mold. Wrap the other ends of the wicks around sticks resting across the top of the mold.

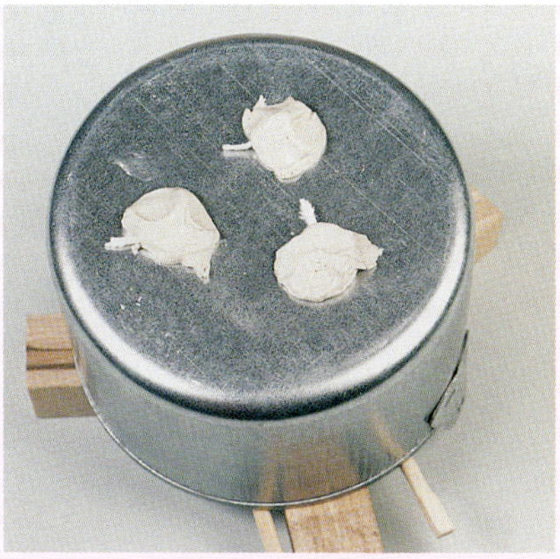

2 Use mold seal to hold the wick ends underneath the mold and to seal the holes securely to make the mold completely watertight. The wicks should be held tight and straight in the mold.

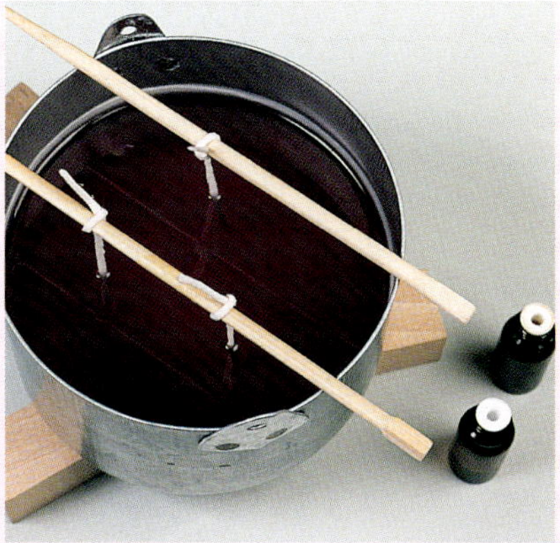

3 Melt the stearin and dye together in a double boiler, then add the wax. Melt and heat the wax mixture to 200°F, then add the perfume. Pour the molten wax into the mold, leaving some wax in the pan to fill it up later.

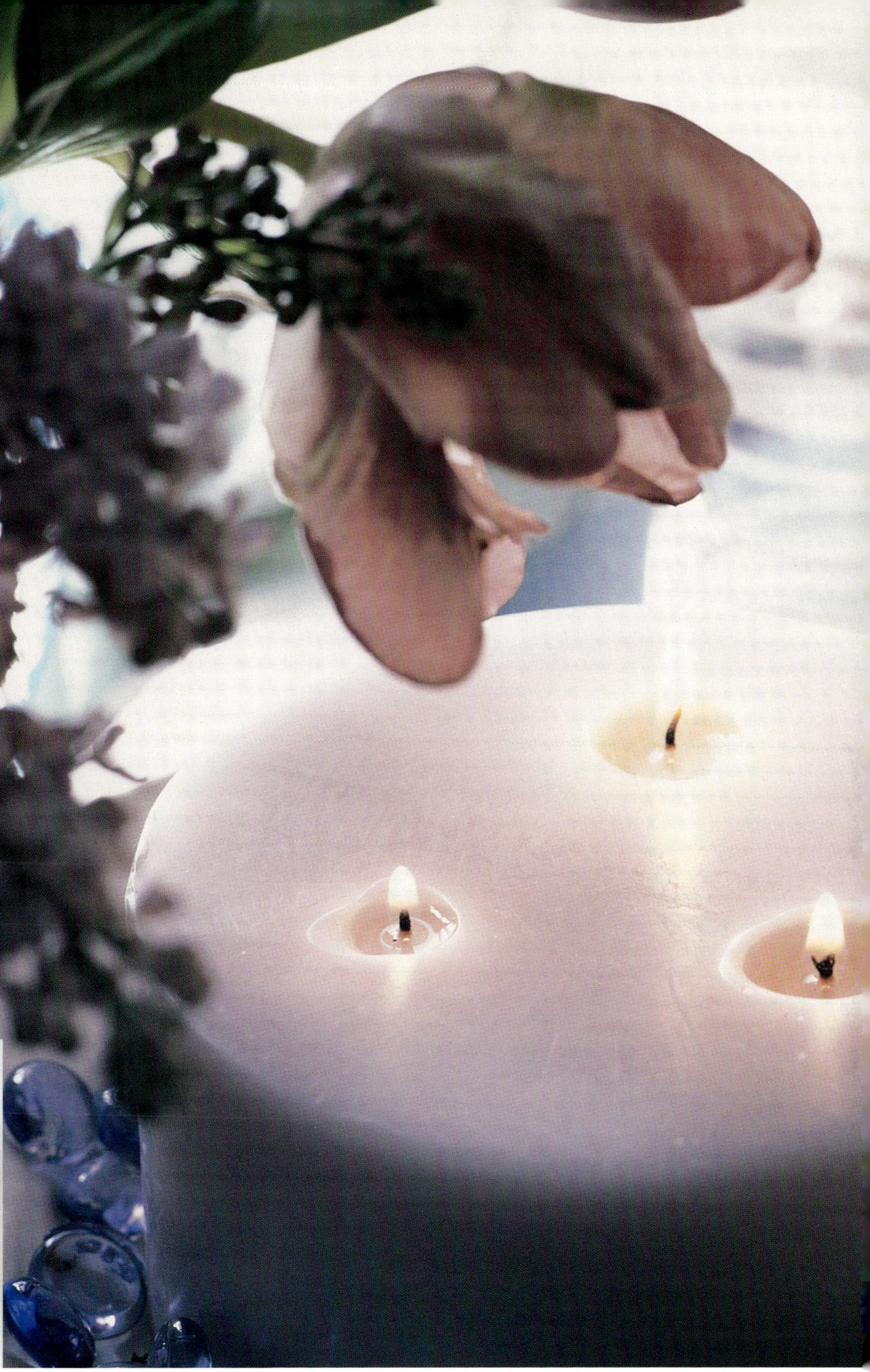

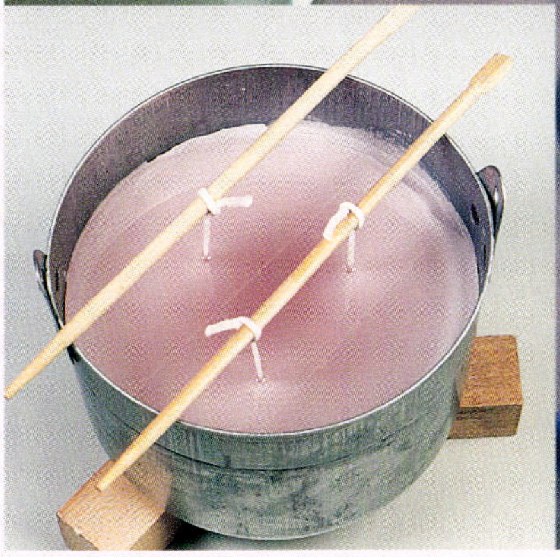

4 Allow the wax to set—craters will form around the wicks as the wax shrinks. Reheat the wax in the pan and fill the craters, taking care that no wax runs down between the candle and the mold. Allow it to cool completely. Carefully remove from the mold and trim the wicks.

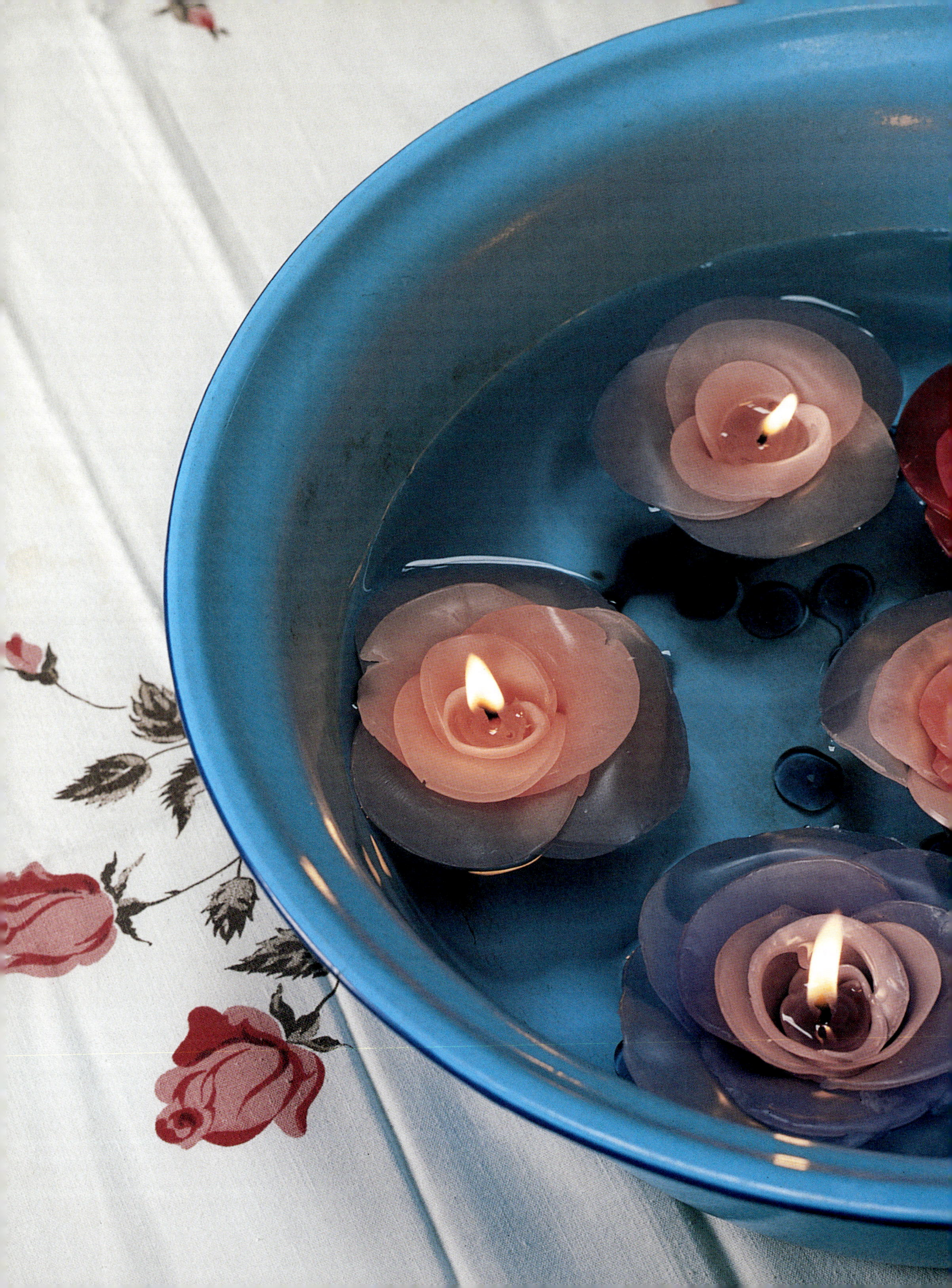

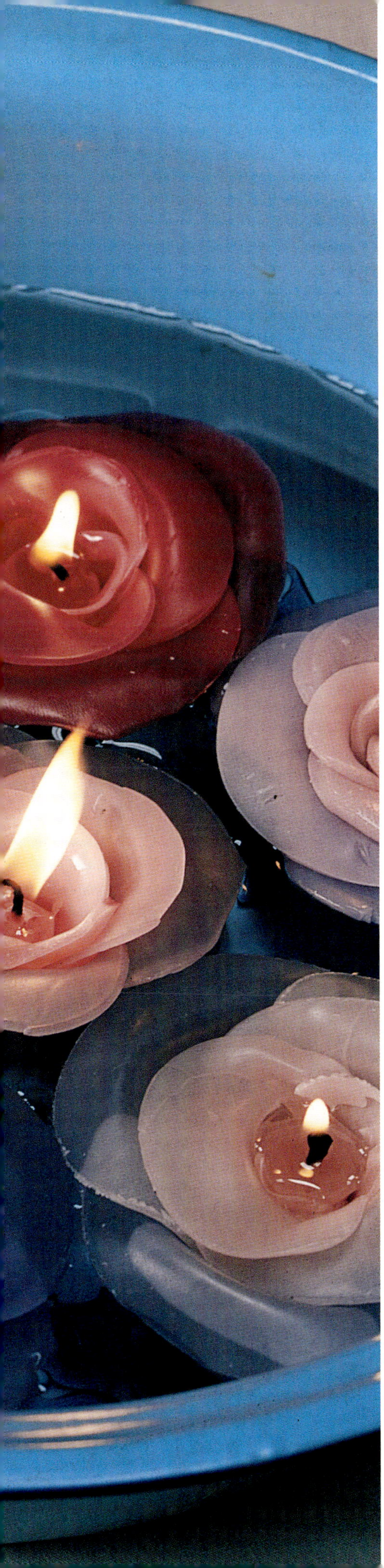

Mauve glass nuggets peek through from beneath the floating flowers, complementing the transparent nature of the display. The nuggets glint magically when the light from the flames catches them. Each rose candle will burn for approximately one hour.

rose floating candles

A cottage garden with rambling roses and deliciously scented blooms overflowing from herbaceous borders is a classic image associated with summer. Roses appear in a profusion of varieties and colors, from the gathered petals of old country roses to the fleeting single-flowered species roses and the crisper lines of formal hybrid teas. Even though we carry with us an idea of how a rose should smell, each variety possesses its own particular fragrance.

Floating candles have a mesmerizing quality as they slowly move around, reflecting the light of the flames on the mirrored surface of the water. A bowl of floating scented candles makes a sensational table centerpiece. Use colored glass nuggets in the base of the bowl and float real leaves among the blooms as a finishing touch.

These rose candles are formed petal by petal, so each one looks individual. The petals are cut from a thin wax sheet, then wrapped and folded to form the flower. As only enough wax for one flower is melted at a time, you can dye it into a range of close shades. Leftover wax can be melted again and reused. Pure rose oil is one of the most expensive oils, taking up to 60,000 blooms to extract just ½ oz. of essential rose oil, known as "rose otto" or "absolute," but there are good synthetic versions, some created especially for candle making.

you will need:

4½ oz. dip-and-carve wax
Wax dye
Approximately 1 tsp. essential oil or wax perfume
Primed medium wick
Marble slab or nonstick baking sheet

MAKING THE CANDLES A marble slab is the only special equipment needed, but a nonstick baking sheet also works. To prevent wax from sticking to the marble, wet it well before pouring on the layer of wax. The temperature of the room will make a difference in how the wax will handle. If it hardens too fast and becomes brittle, warm it with a blast of heat from a hair dryer to restore malleability. It is important to check that the finished flower will float. If water starts to seep through the flower, dip its base in molten wax to seal any gaps between the petals. For the longest burning time, the flower center should stand slightly proud of the outer petals. Dip-and-carve wax is used, as it is more malleable than paraffin wax. Each rose measures about ½ inch across.

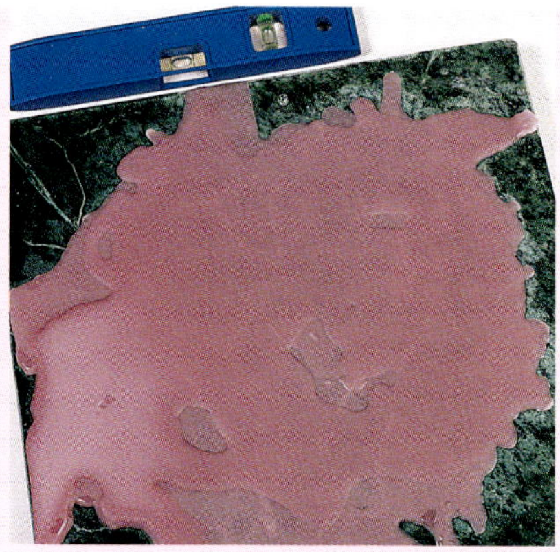

1 Make sure your table surface is level. Melt the wax in a small pan and add the dye. Heat the wax to 180°F. Thoroughly wet the surface of a marble slab, then pour the wax onto the marble, working from the center outward, so the wax is slightly thicker at the center and becoming thinner toward the edges.

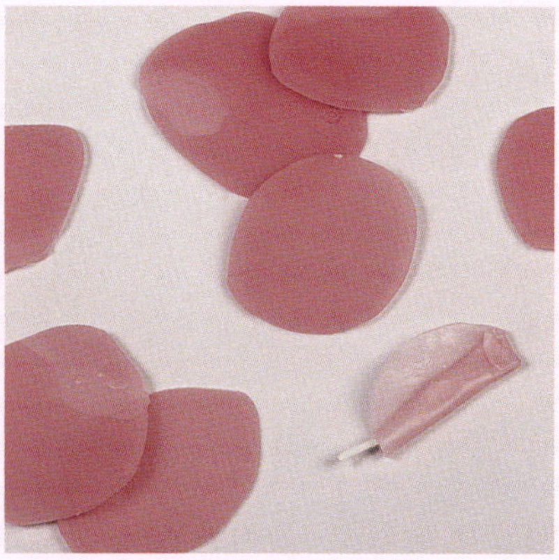

3 Cut the wick into a 2–3 inch length, then roll a petal tightly around the wick to form the rose center, leaving ¾ inch of wick sticking out of the top end and folding the wax over at the other end.

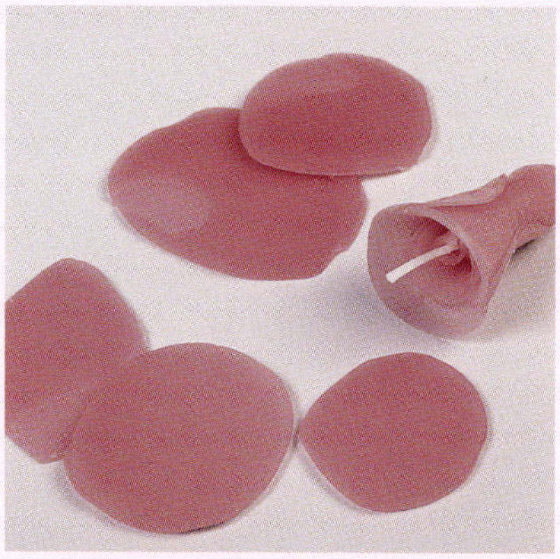

4 One by one, wrap the other petals around the flower center, folding back the wax shapes to give a natural look to the flower and staggering the placement of the petals as you go.

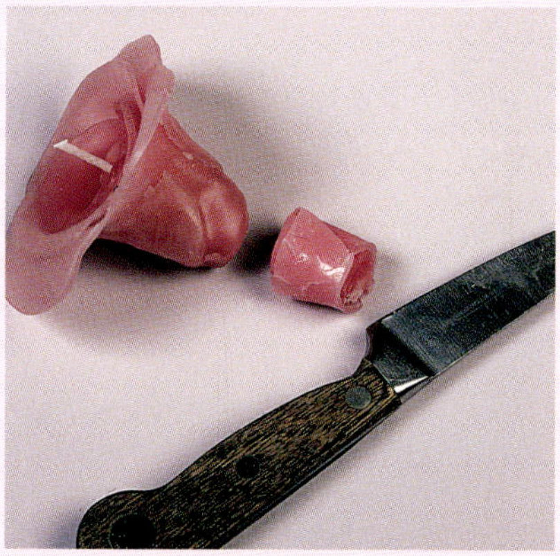

5 If the wax becomes too cold and unworkable, warm it with the heat from a hair dryer to make the wax malleable again. When all the petals are in place, trim the flower's base with a knife.

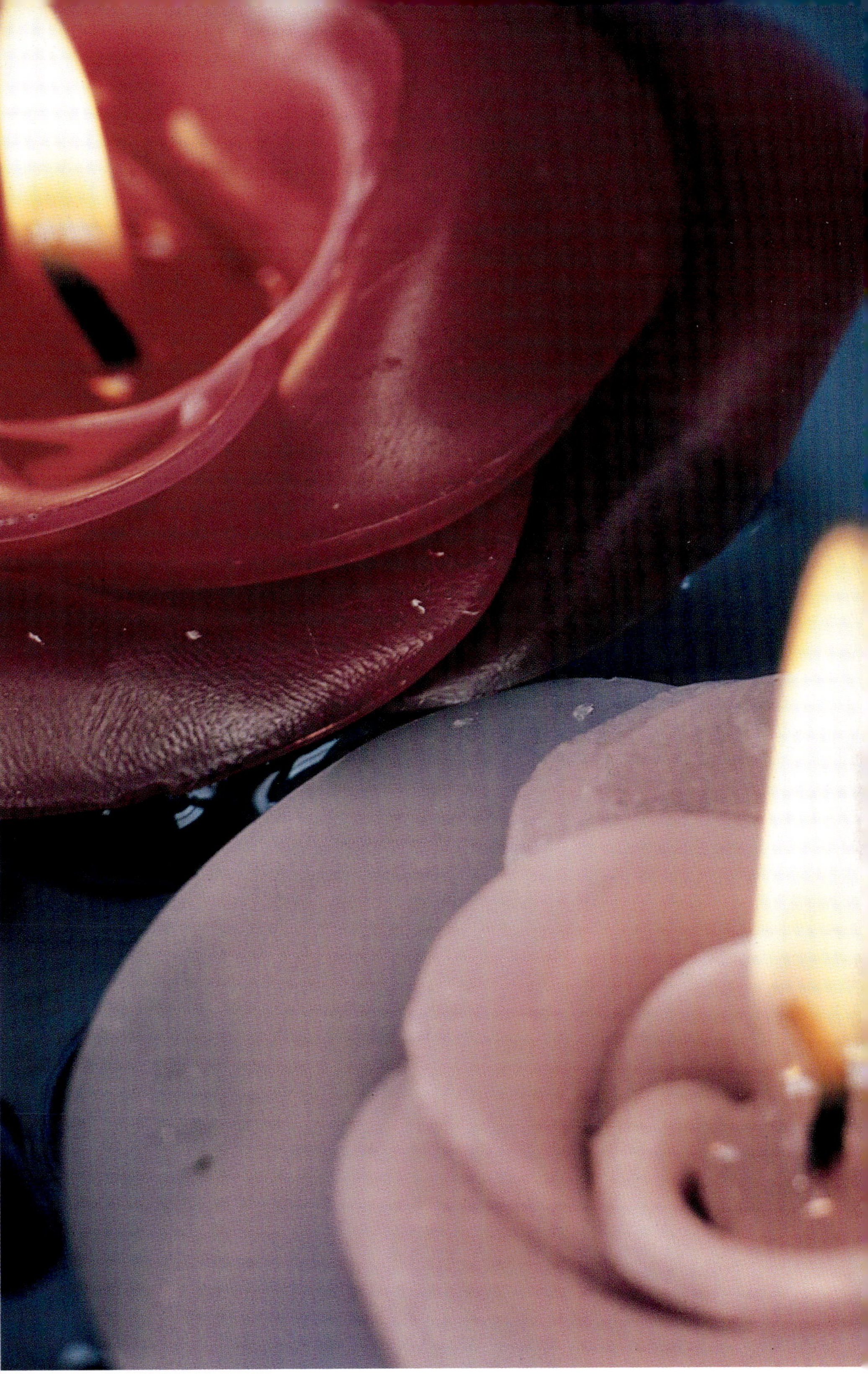

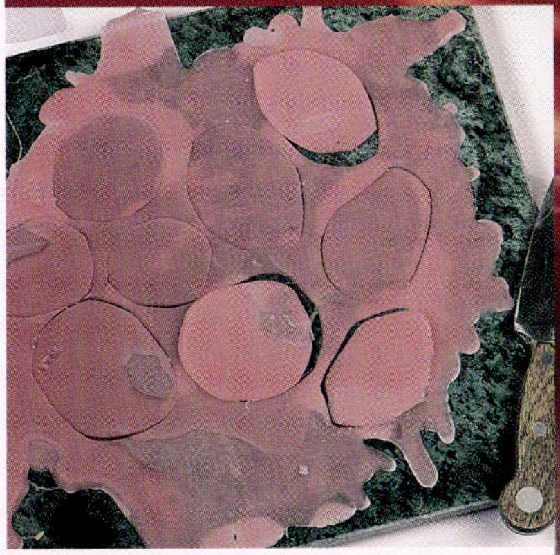

2 Let the wax cool and set slightly so it feels rubbery. Using a sharp knife and working while the wax is still warm, cut out rough circles for the petals, making them different sizes. You will need approximately eight petals for each rose.

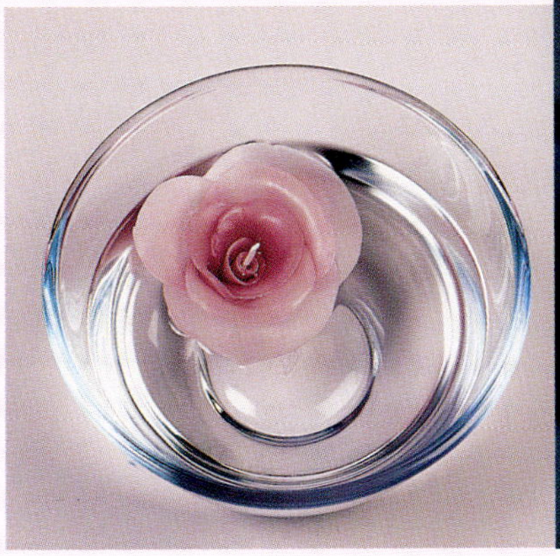

6 Test to see if the flower will float evenly without any water seeping up between the petals by floating it in a bowl of water. If water seeps through, dip the candle base in melted wax to seal any gaps.

Large outdoor candles can be costly to buy but, like all container candles, are straightforward to make. Amazingly stylish, this monochrome concrete planter filled with scented white wax and roomy enough to accommodate several wicks makes a bold, modern statement and provides illumination in the garden as the sun goes down. Spicy and calming, black pepper and bergamot create an unusual yet sensuous combination to scent a porch or patio. Alternatively, choose heady floral scents to enhance the fragrances of surrounding garden plants, which are at their best at dusk or, on a practical note, opt for citronella oil to discourage mosquitoes from biting bare arms and ankles.

outdoor candles

you will need:

- Concrete planter
- Mold sealant
- Prepared container wick
- 4 wick sustainers
- 14 lb. paraffin wax
- Approximately 2 fl. oz. essential oil or candle perfume

MAKING THE CANDLE First, make sure the container is watertight. Block any holes in the base using mold seal or a special waterproof sealant from a hardware store. The combination of a large pot and the quantity of wax needed to fill it does produce a weighty candle that can be heavy to move, so take care when positioning it. Also consider carefully where it should go so that it doesn't create a hazard for people walking by or energetic children running around. The candle is big enough to give many hours of burning time. For this amount of wax, melt the wax in smaller batches rather than all at once and pour into the planter in layers. To be economical with the perfume, just scent the top third of the wax. This concrete planter measures 10 inches in diameter and 10 inches high.

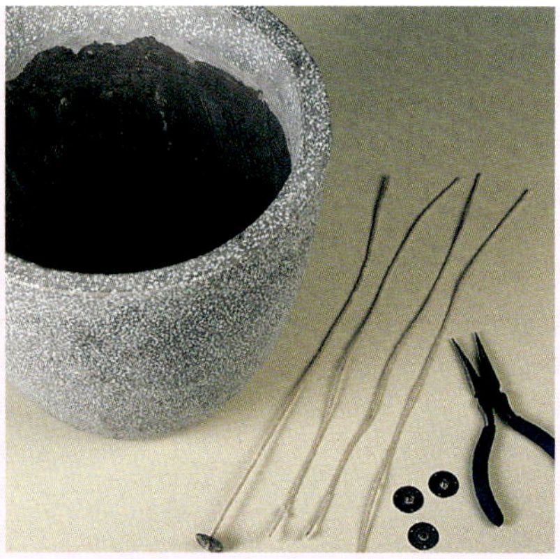

1 Choose a planter without a hole in the base or fill the drainage holes with waterproof putty. Cut the prepared wick into four lengths to the depth of the planter, plus a little extra. Fix a wick sustainer to one end of each wick, securing with pliers.

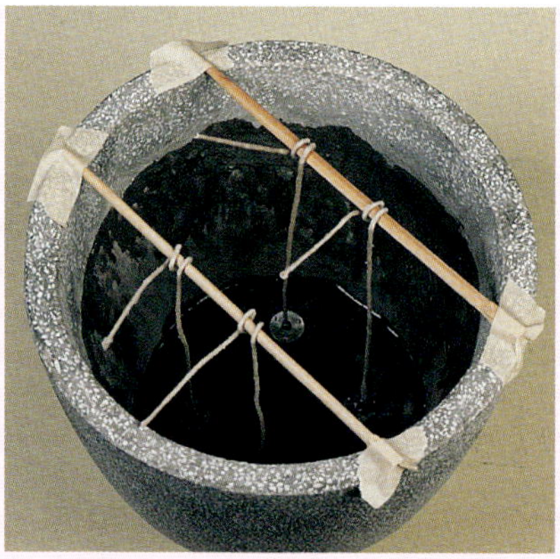

2 Place the wicks in position, equally spaced inside the planter with the wick sustainers resting on the base. Use wicking needles or sticks held in place with masking tape to provide supports for the wicks.

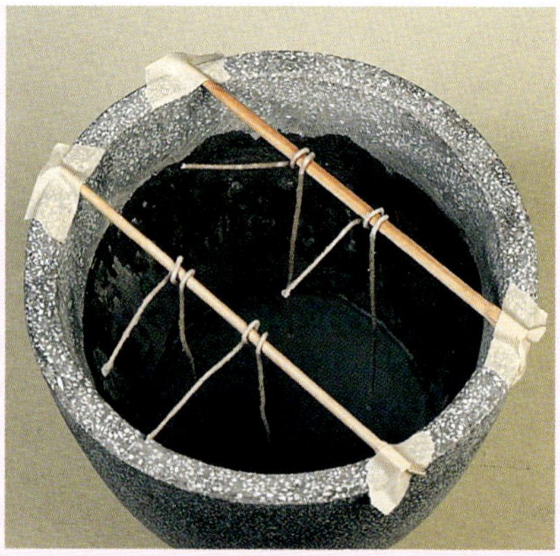

3 Melt the paraffin wax, then add the oil or perfume as required. Heat to 160°F. Pour a shallow layer of melted wax into the planter base and allow it to set to hold the wicks. Fill the planter with melted wax to within 1½ inches of the rim, pouring carefully to keep the rim clear of splashes. Allow the wax to set and shrink down in the center.

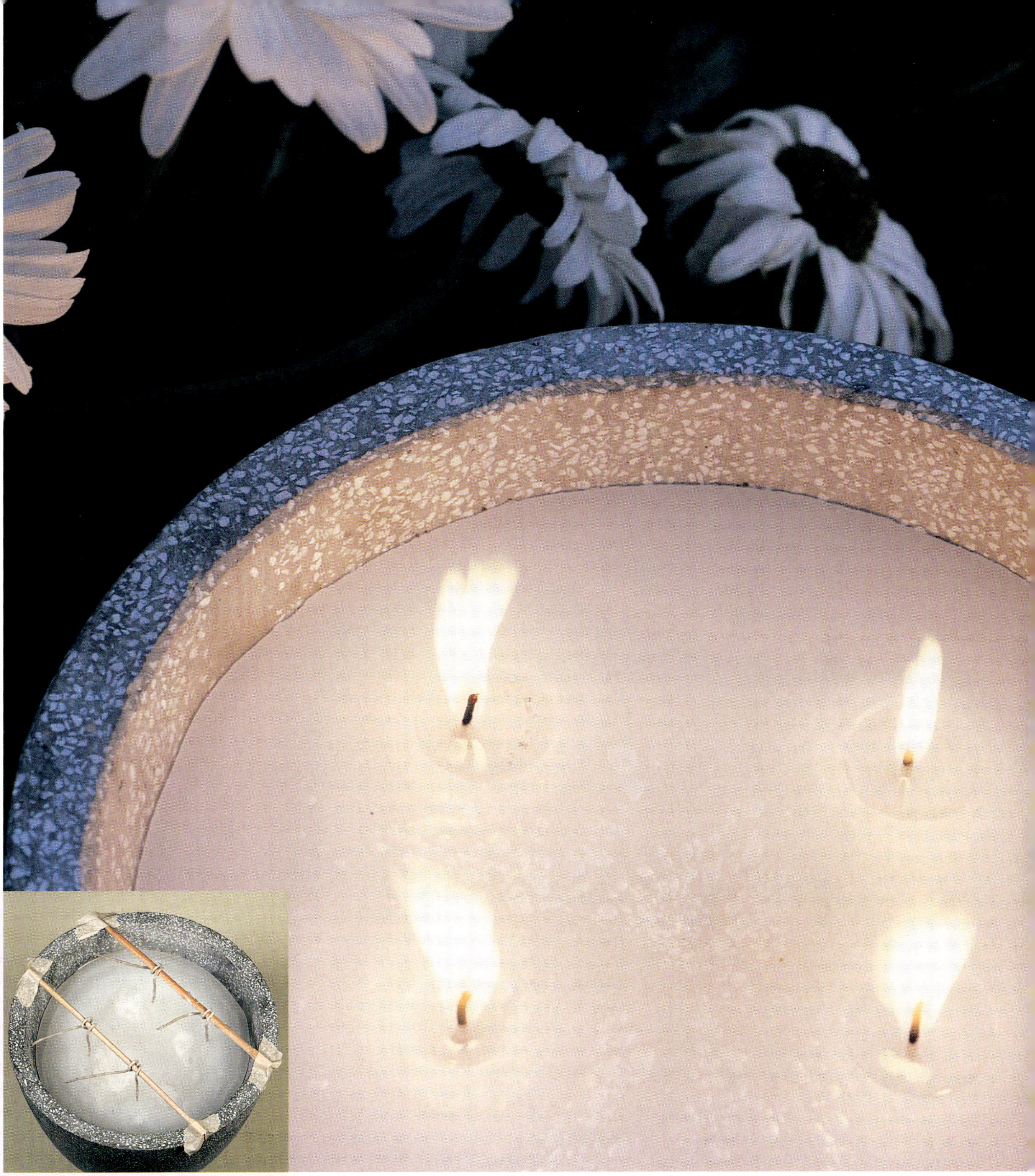

4 Fill the craters that form around the wicks on the candle's surface with more molten wax to make it level, then allow to set. When the wax is completely cold, remove the wicking needles and trim the wicks to 1 inch.

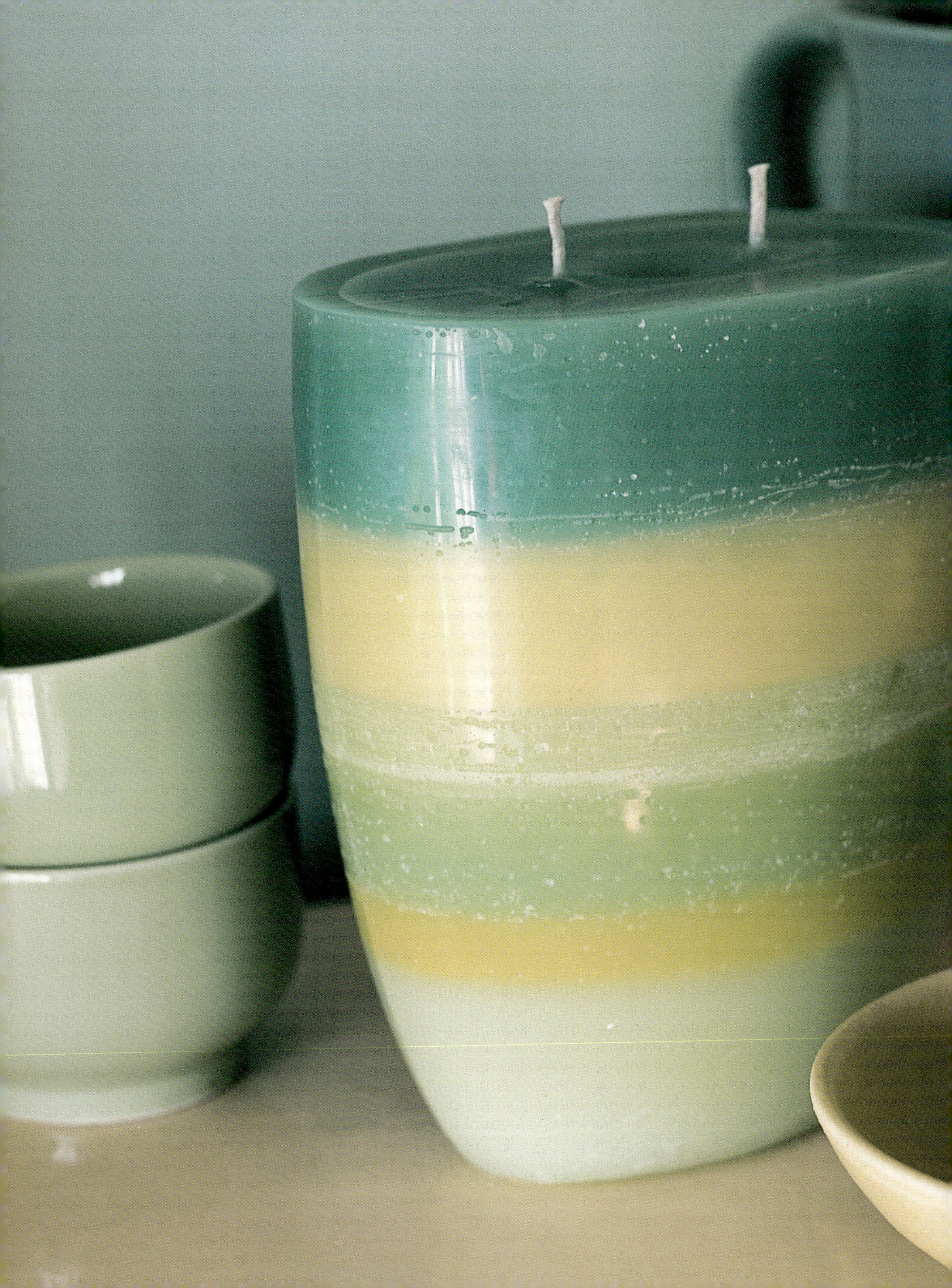

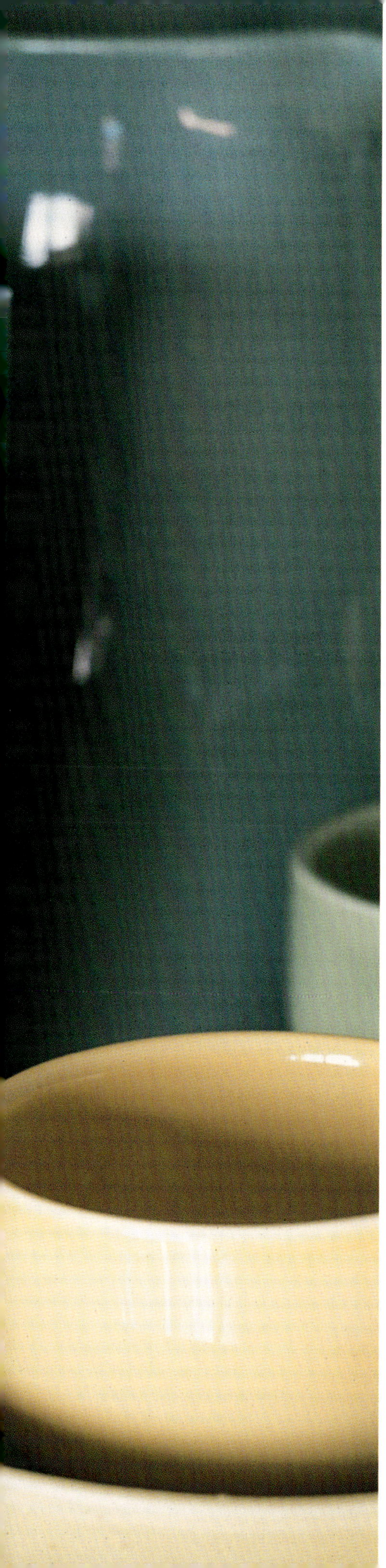

Different shades within a restricted color range work well, as do stripes of varying thicknesses. They also show the contrasting textures created by pouring the wax at different temperatures.

striped candles

Stripes in design are classic and reliable, always seeming to work whether woven together in traditional ticking stripes or used in modern, youthful combinations of thick and thin lines in the style of bar codes. For a striped candle, the separate, random bands of color in different widths give a look that is confident and contemporary. By using single scents in each stripe, the fragrance changes as the candle burns down, and each different scent has a chance to shine through and dominate. A fresh and fruity combination, the lively, uplifting scents of grapefruit, mandarin, and lime work well together but also succeed when standing alone. The candle smells wonderful as it burns but also looks fabulously stylish unlit.

Unusual shaped molds can make a homemade candle unique. An oval glass vase that is wider at the top than the base is an ideal mold for candle making, but watch for bumps on the inner surface which can make it difficult to remove the candle. Also be sure that the base inside is flat or the candle will not sit steady. Remove any uneven lumps on the base by melting the wax with a hot iron. Keeping the colors within a particular hue gives stylish results, or let your creativity run riot with bands of different, contrasting colors.

you will need:

Prepared medium wick
Wick sustainers
Suitable mold
7 oz. stearin
Wax dyes
2½ lb. paraffin wax beads
Approximately 2¼ fl. oz. essential oil or wax perfume

MAKING THE CANDLE A striped candle is a great way to use up leftover wax. Similar shades can be mixed to create a vibrant palette, but mixing contrasting colors at random can create exciting results. Allow a drop of any mixed molten wax to cool to see the color when cold. When making the stripes, the trick is gauging the right time to pour on a new layer. Let each stripe of wax cool before adding the next. The surface of the stripe beneath needs to form a skin and be soft and rubbery but not set. The amount of wax, stearin, and perfume shown is for the whole candle. When melting smaller quantities for stripes, use 20 percent stearin and 5 percent perfume to the amount of wax. This candle measures 6 by 3 inches at the top and is 6 inches high.

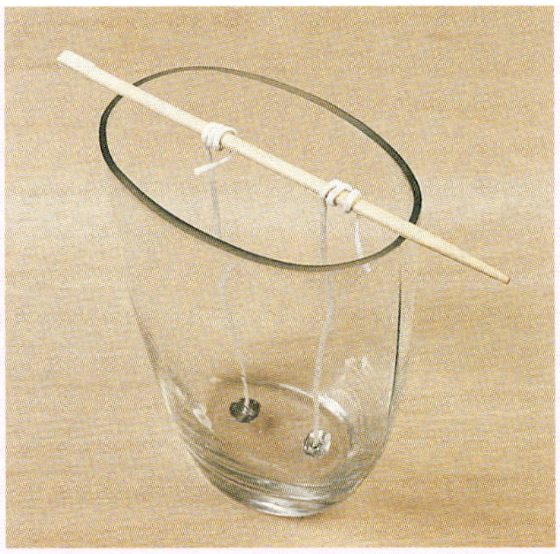

1 Cut two lengths of wick to the depth of the container plus a little extra. Attach wick sustainers to one end of each wick, squeezing the metal shut with pliers to secure. Place the wicks in the mold with the sustainers on the base, wrapping the extra wick around a stick to hold it steady.

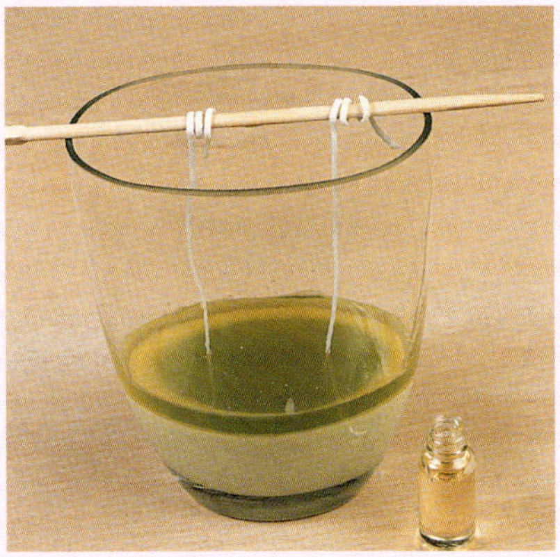

3 Following the guidelines given above, allowing a skin to form on the stripe below before pouring on the next, begin to build up the candle in random stripes. Place the mold in a water bath to cool the candle faster.

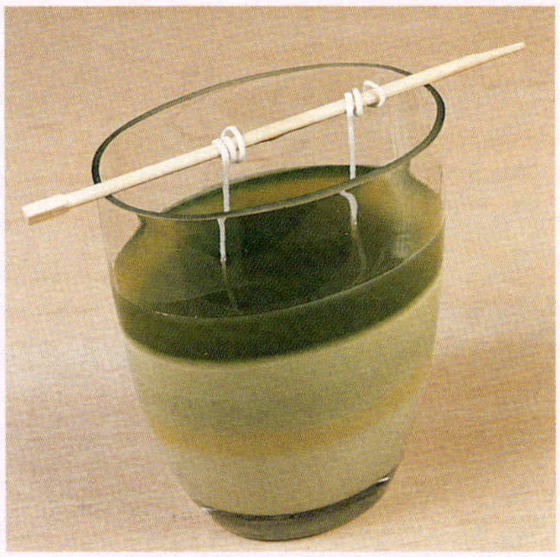

4 Pour each layer with care so the molten wax doesn't burst through into the layer below and liquid wax doesn't splash onto the mold. Do not allow the candle to cool too much or it will shrink away from the sides of the mold before the next stripe is poured in.

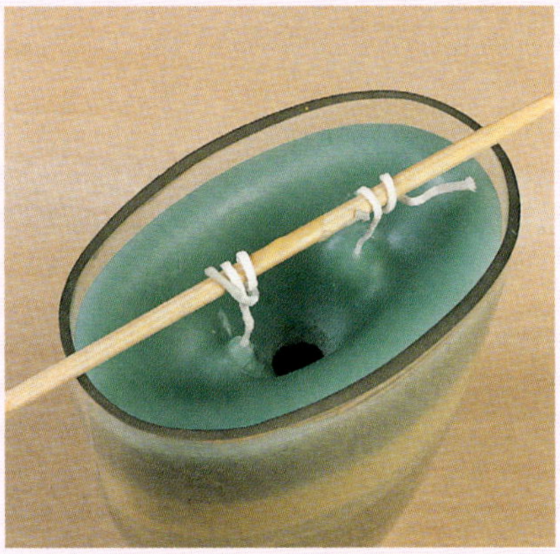

5 After pouring in the last stripe, allow the candle to cool completely, saving some wax in the final stripe color in the pan. As the wax cools and shrinks, cavities will appear around the wick.

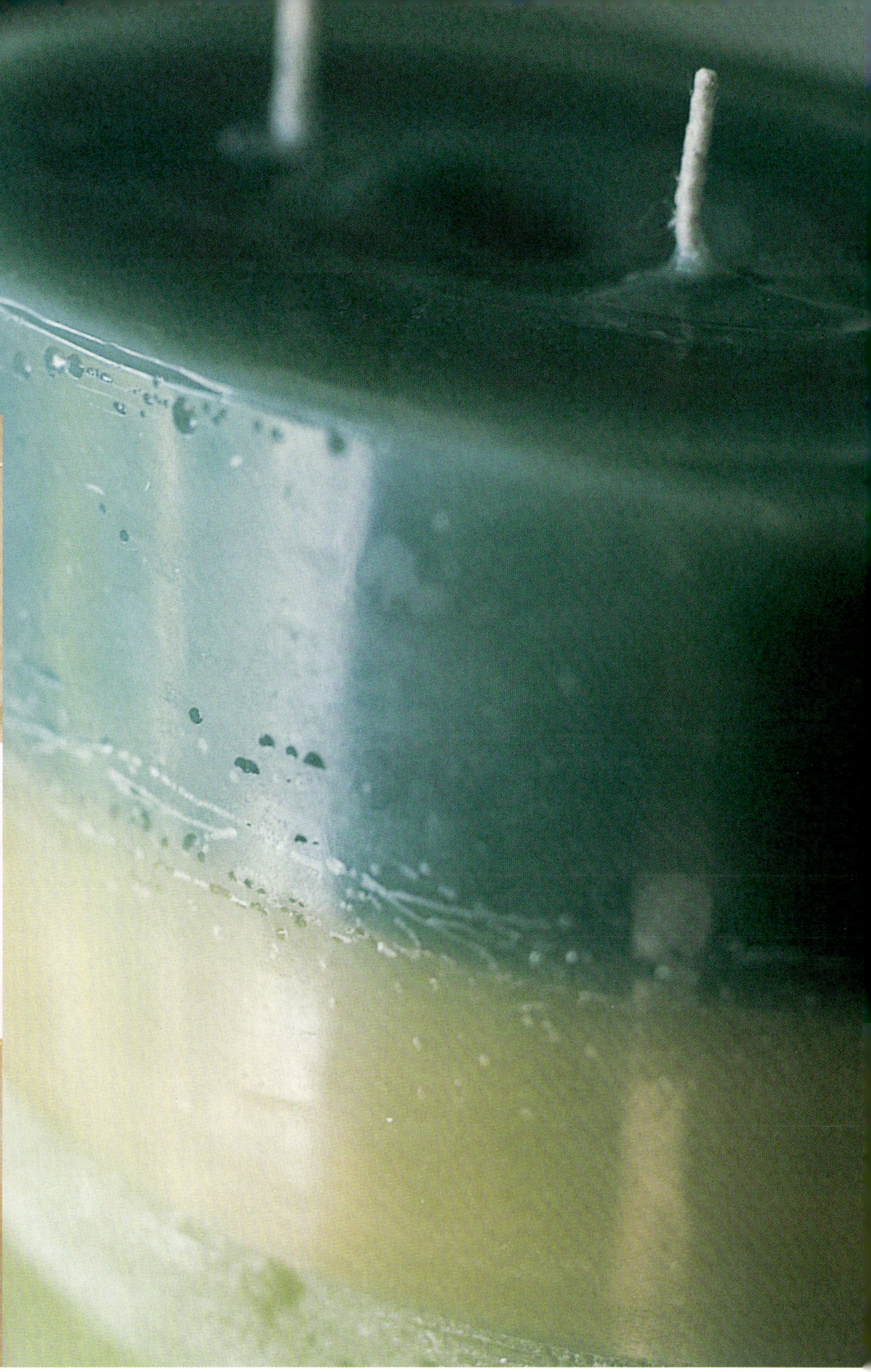

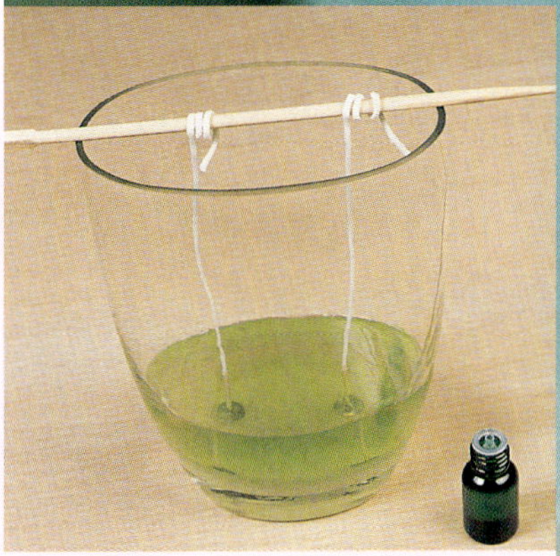

2 Melt the stearin and dye together, then add the paraffin wax. Alternatively, melt together bits of leftover wax. For smooth, flat, colored stripes, heat the wax to 200°F, or for a more textured surface heat to only 160°F—or combine the two textures. Add the perfume and pour the first stripe into the mold.

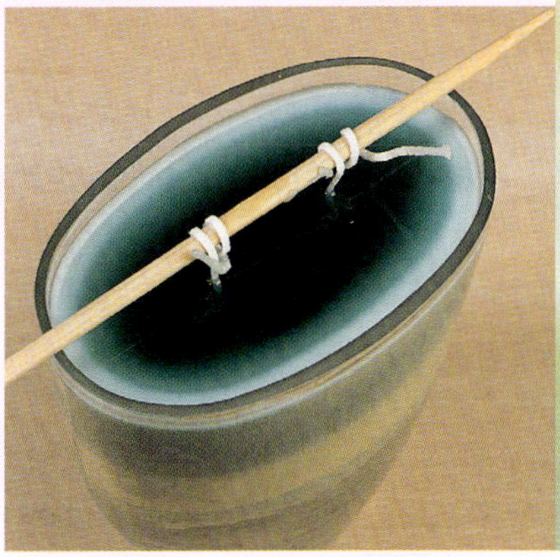

6 Reheat the remaining wax in the pan and fill the cavity that has formed, taking care that no molten wax runs down between the mold and the candle. Allow to cool completely, then remove the candle from the mold and trim the wick.

Small floating rose candles, all made individually in a range of rosy pink shades, capture the true essence of summer.

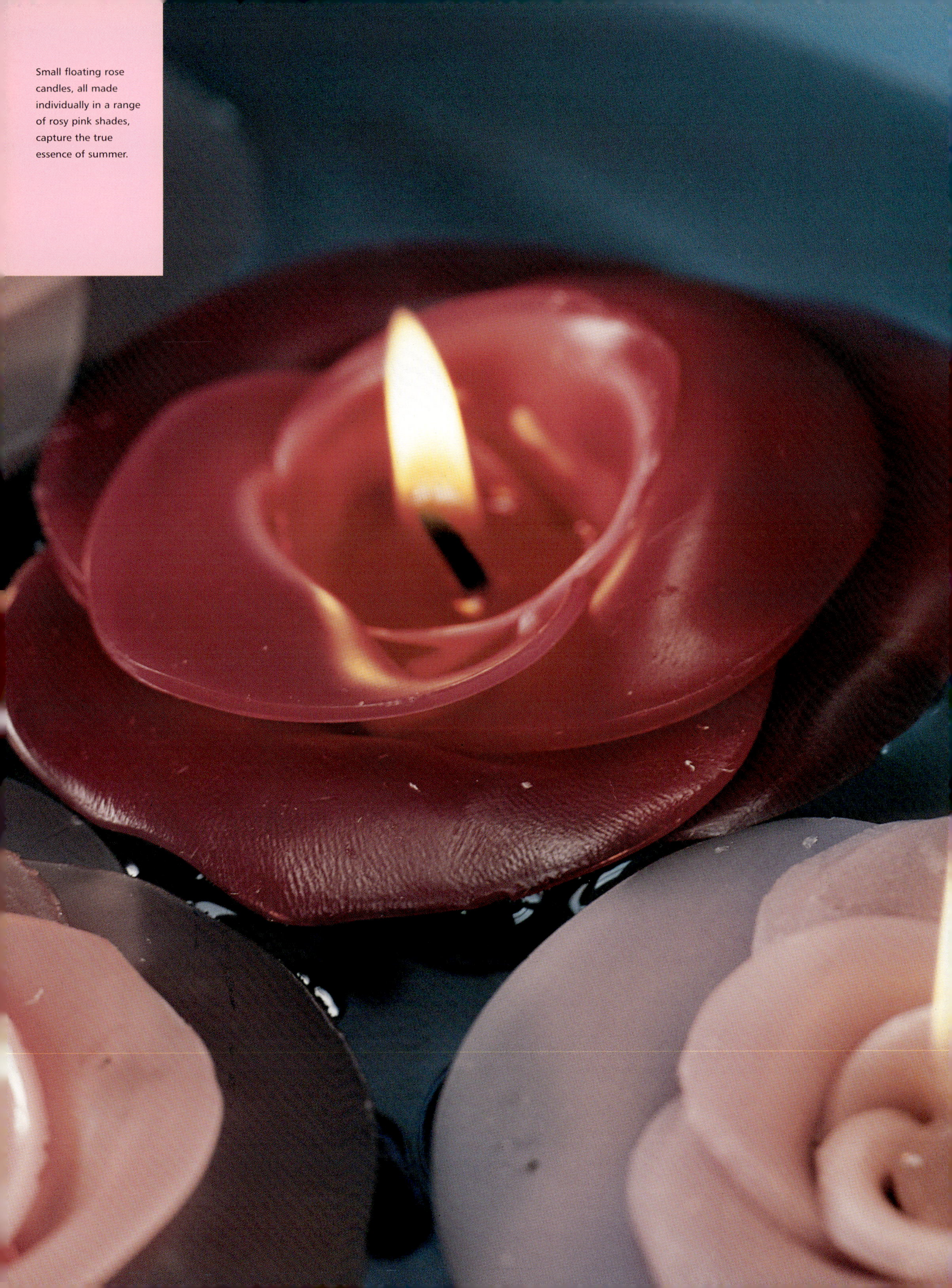

SUMMER COLORS

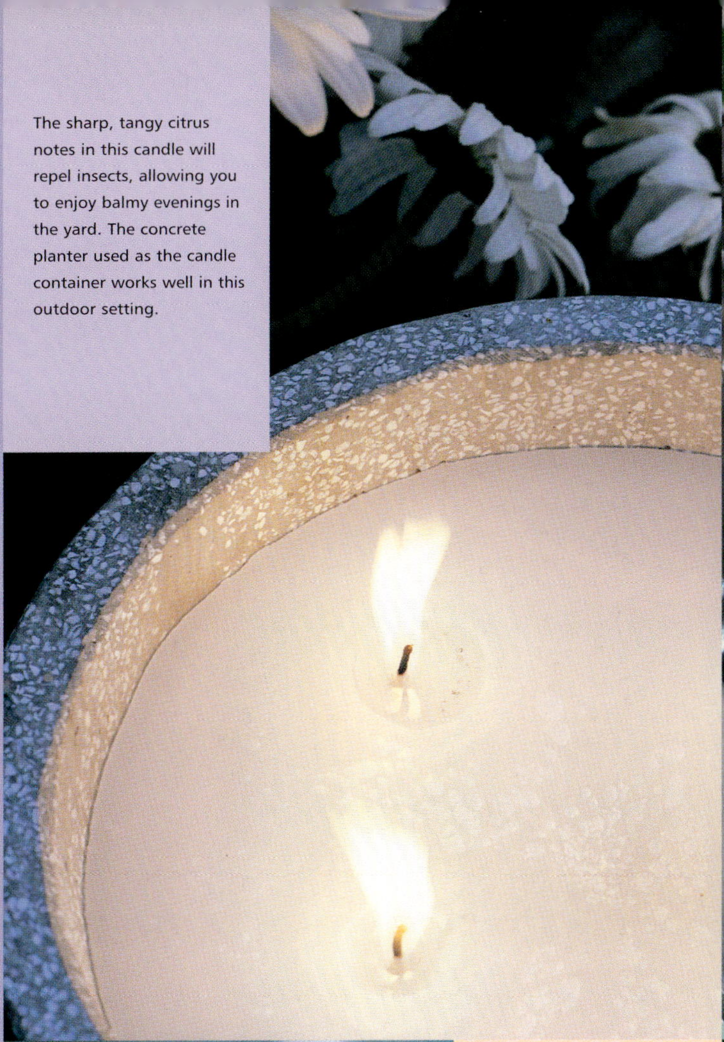

The sharp, tangy citrus notes in this candle will repel insects, allowing you to enjoy balmy evenings in the yard. The concrete planter used as the candle container works well in this outdoor setting.

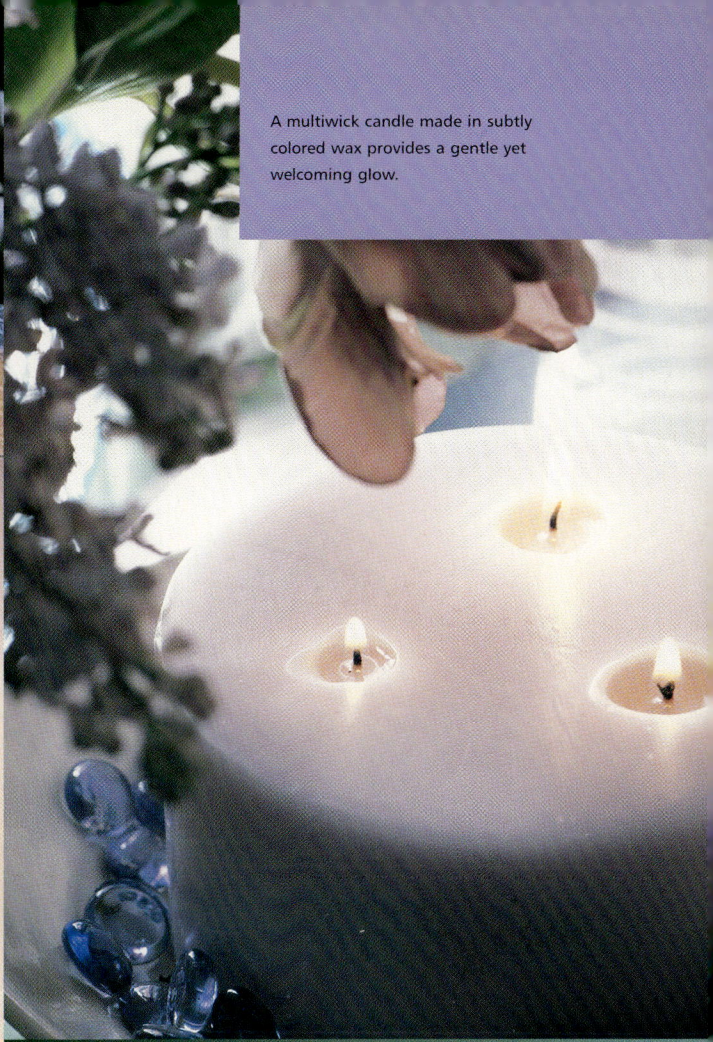

A multiwick candle made in subtly colored wax provides a gentle yet welcoming glow.

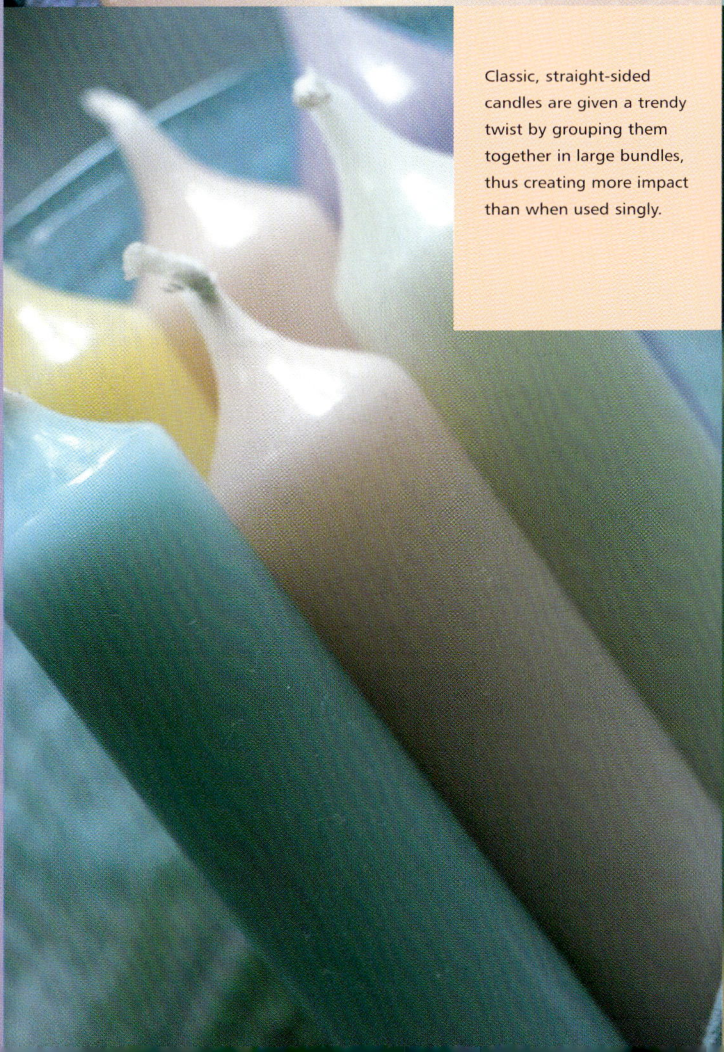

Classic, straight-sided candles are given a trendy twist by grouping them together in large bundles, thus creating more impact than when used singly.

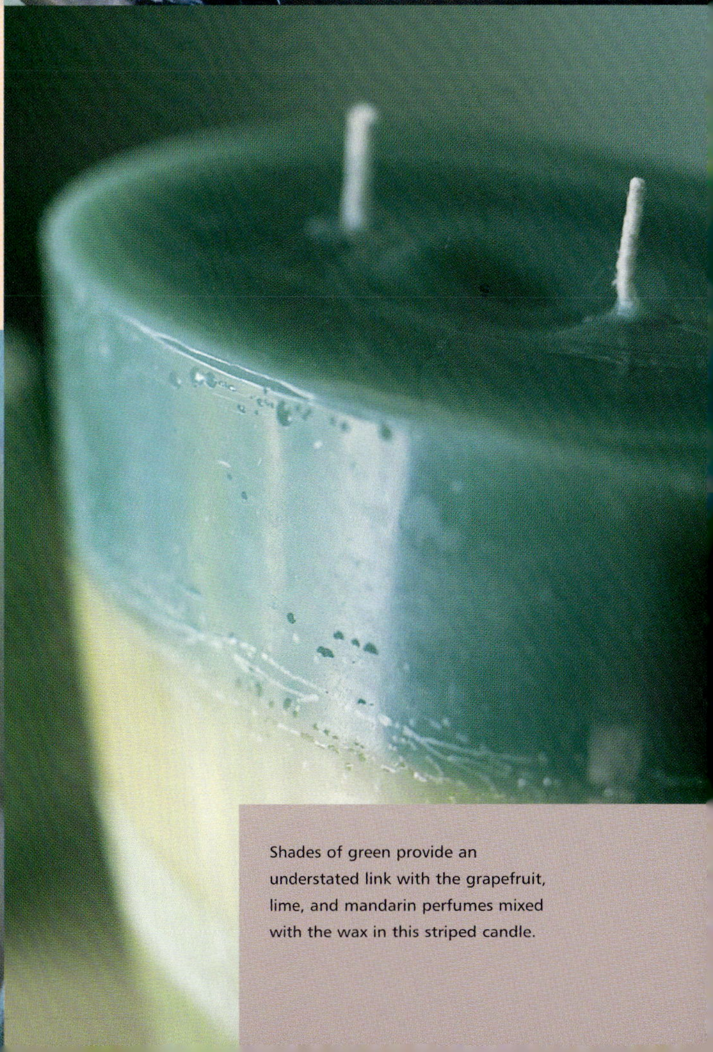

Shades of green provide an understated link with the grapefruit, lime, and mandarin perfumes mixed with the wax in this striped candle.

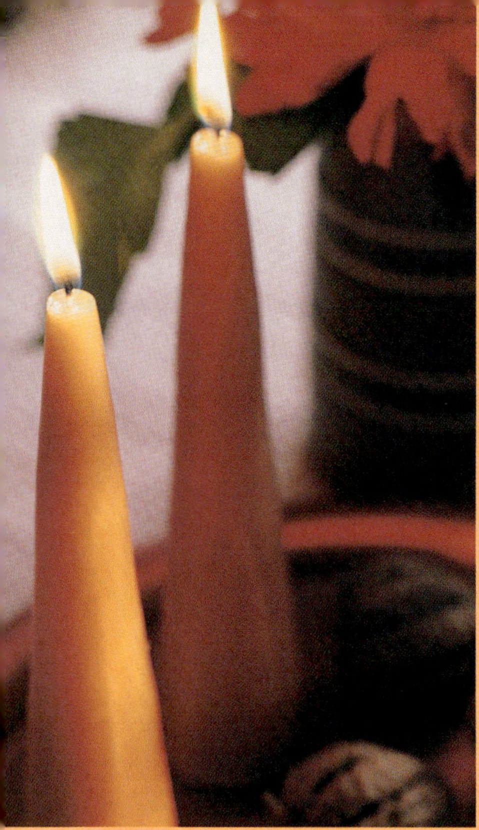

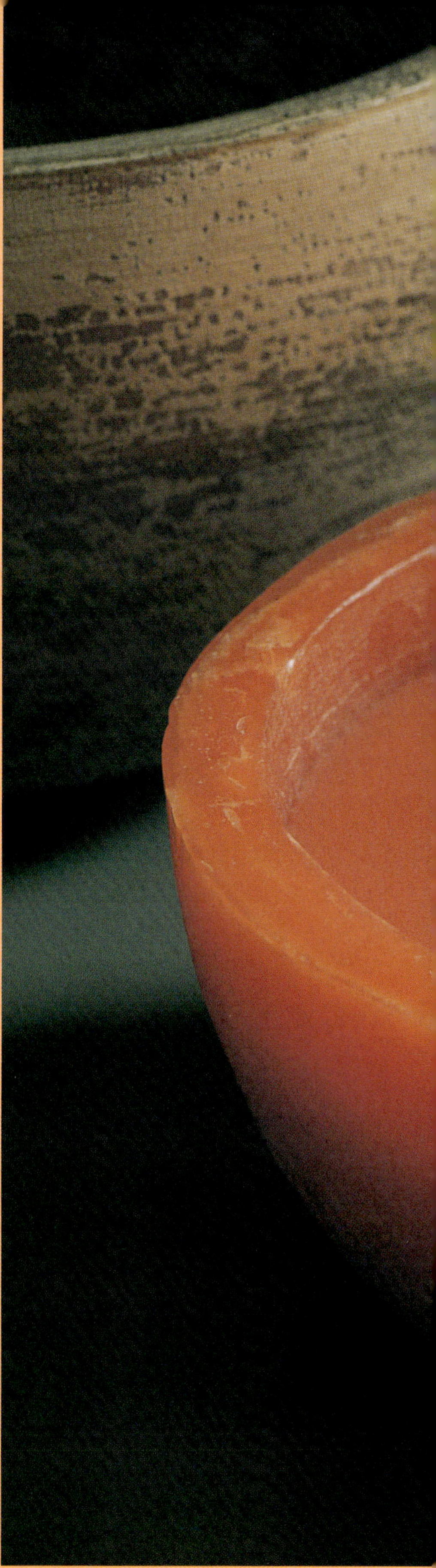

ESSENCE OF fall

As the leaves on the trees change color and flutter to the ground, the final fruits of summer are safely gathered in. Now is the time to retreat into the warmth and comfort of home. Even as the hours of daylight lessen, there is still much to lift the spirits and excite the senses. Fallen leaves surround us in uplifting shades of amber, crimson, chestnut, and burnished copper. Colorful dahlias and wild asters add their rich colors to the fall palette. Candlelight comes into its own, bringing magic to the gloom of a dark afternoon and creating a warming atmosphere in the evening. Choose positive and comforting fragrances to create a sanctuary against the changeable elements.

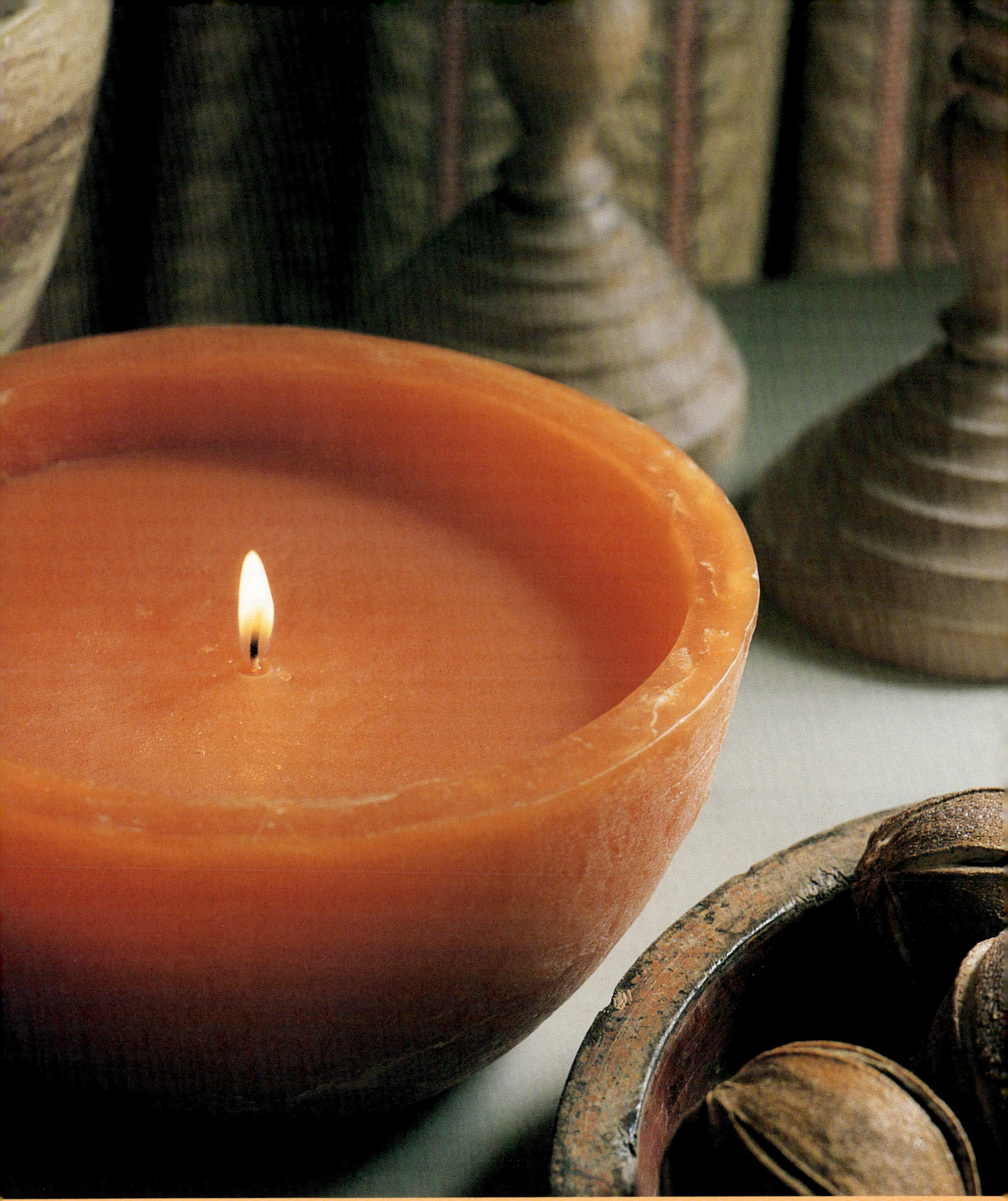

Echoing the uplifting shades of the season, as seen in burnished leaves and vibrant pumpkins, a candle brings a warming glow to lift the spirits.

The deep green wax used for this candle echoes its botanical influences and is scented with warm sandalwood, nutmeg, and black pepper. As the candle burns down, trim away any part of the leaf that stands above the edge to prevent it from catching on fire. Use flat, dry leaves and petals that can curve around the candle's surface—dried skeleton leaves create a subtle, embossed effect. To fix in place, heat a metal teaspoon in boiling water, then run the back of the spoon over the leaf to make the wax sticky. Move the spoon in a circular motion, holding it still on the leaf's edge for an extra secure bond.

leaf candle

you will need:

- Pillar candle mold
- Prepared wick
- Mold seal
- Wicking needle
- 4½ oz. stearin
- Wax dye
- 1 lb. paraffin wax beads
- 1 fl. oz. essential oil or wax perfume
- Dried skeleton leaf
- Metal teaspoon
- Dipping can and paraffin wax

MAKING THE CANDLE After fixing the leaf in place on the candle with a hot spoon, it is necessary to dip the candle with a couple of fine layers of wax to seal the decoration and keep it from lifting off. To test how long to dip the candle for, prepare a spare candle and a leaf in exactly the same manner. Heat enough white paraffin wax in a dipping can to 200°F so the candle will be completely submerged when dipped into it, then dip the spare candle in the wax, counting the seconds until the leaf falls off—this should take about 8–9 seconds. Dip the actual candle, holding it in the wax for 1 second less than it took for the leaf to separate from the test candle. Allow to cool, making sure any bits of leaf that have come away are pushed back into position. When the wax begins to clear but is still warm, dip the whole thing again for 3 seconds. This will securely laminate the leaf in place. This mold measures 3½ inches in diameter and 5 inches high.

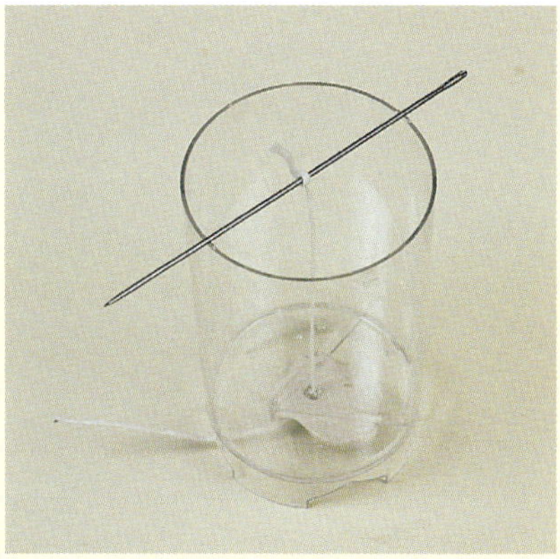

1 Prepare the mold by threading the wick through the base. Seal the hole with mold seal to make it watertight. Place a wicking needle across the top of the mold and tie the other end of the wick to it tightly.

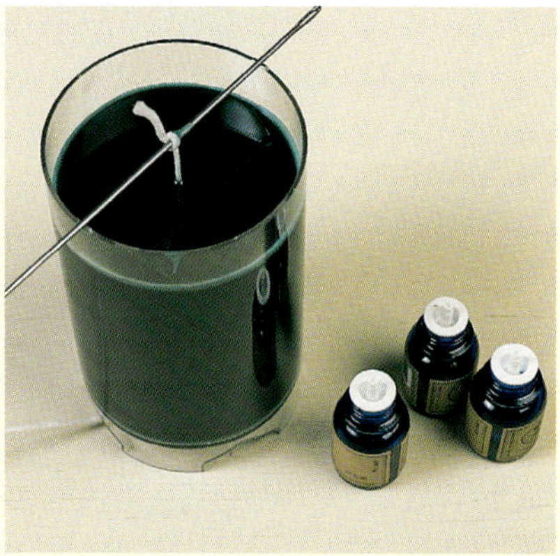

2 Melt the stearin together with the dye in the top of a double boiler, then add the wax. Melt and heat the mixture to 200°F. Add perfume and mix in, then pour into the prepared mold. To hasten cooling, place in a water bath.

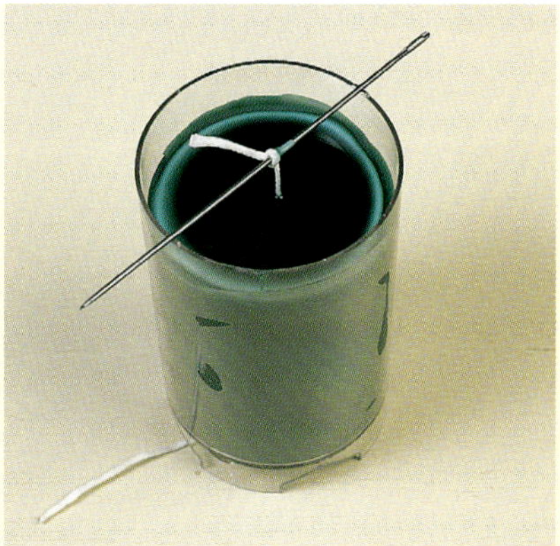

3 When the wax has set, reheat the wax as before and fill the cavities around the wick, taking care that wax doesn't run down between the candle and the mold. Allow to cool completely. Remove from the mold and trim the wick.

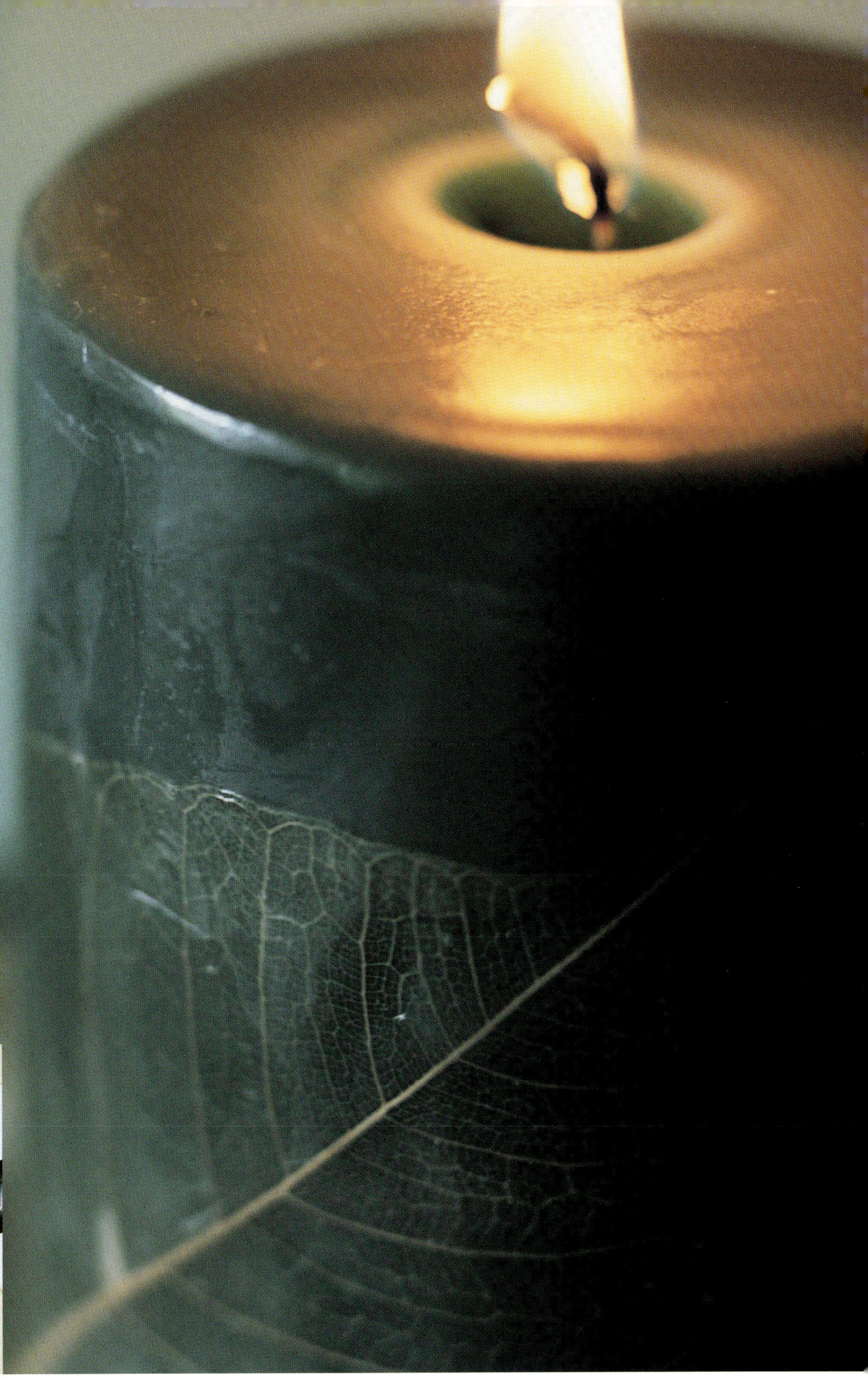

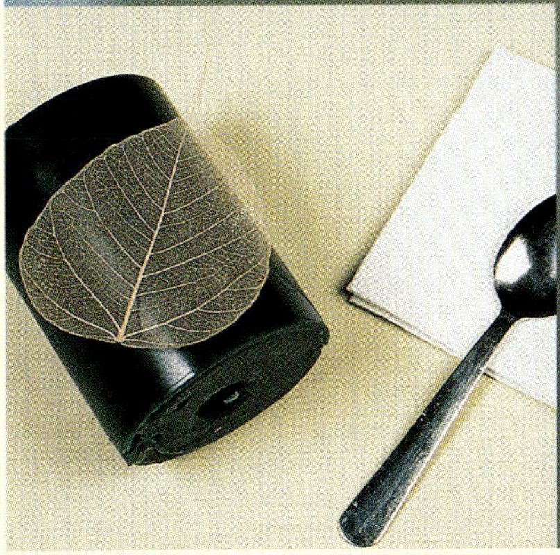

4 Place the leaf in position on the candle and run the back of a hot teaspoon over the leaf, paying particular attention to the edges of the leaf. Using a dipping can filled with white paraffin wax heated to 200°F, dip the candle twice as explained above.

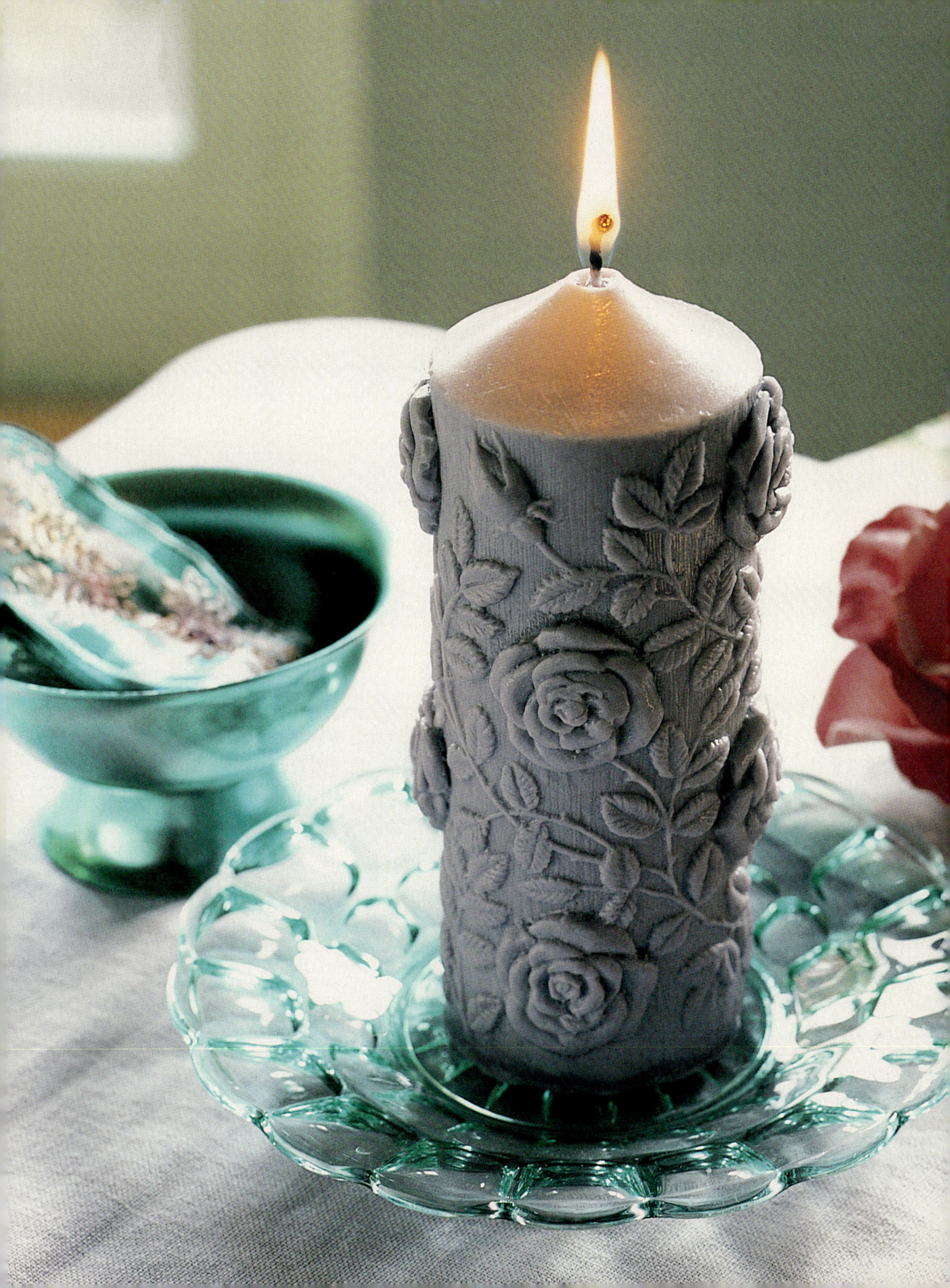

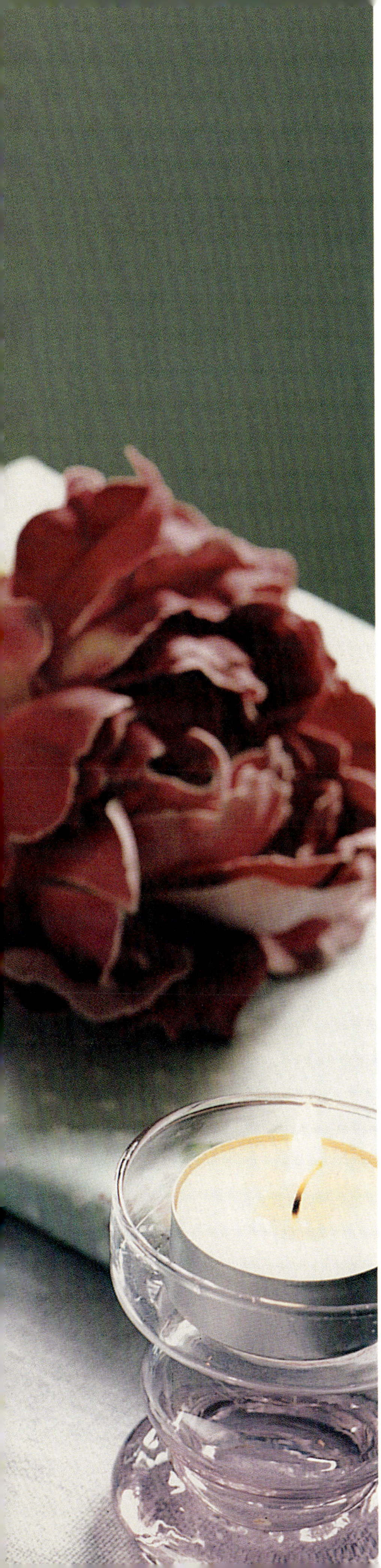

A delicate pattern of briar roses entwines this sumptuous candle and brings a luxurious touch to a room when perfumed with the intoxicating and sensuous blend of rose, vanilla, and patchouli.

embossed candle

The last roses of the year still manage to bloom, even though the feeling of abundance has now passed. Capture these blooms in wax as a reminder in the coming months of the natural habit and fleeting quality of these flowers. A mold richly patterned with twining briar roses creates a magical candle with a fairy-tale quality and looks fabulous displayed with delicate colored glassware. Tight buds and full-blown flowers densely arranged together form an elaborate surface for this pretty candle. Use pure rose oil sparingly, or a less expensive synthetic alternative, to provide a wonderfully powdery note to the perfume, adding the warmth of vanilla and sensuous patchouli to complete the blend.

Rubber molds come in lots of different styles and patterns and can be bought from craft stores. Sumptuously embossed candles can look as if they have cost a fortune but they are surprisingly easy to make. By first pouring in a pale colored wax to coat just the raised motifs, then following this with a deeper shade to provide a contrasting background and core for the candle, the embossed effect produced is two-tone and can be very dramatic. Candle makers refer to this technique as "pour-in pour-out." Here a truly heavenly blend of sensuous rose, vanilla, and patchouli creates a combination that matches the opulence of the ornate briar rose relief.

you will need:

- Rubber mold
- Wick (unprimed)
- Wicking needle
- 20 oz. paraffin wax
- ⅛ oz. Vybar
- Wax dye
- 1 fl. oz. wax perfume
- liquid soap

MAKING THE CANDLE Flexible rubber molds can be used to make highly embossed and decorative candles, as they are removed by peeling them away from the textured surface. Always use unprimed wick with this type of mold in order to limit the size of the hole you make in the mold. When setting up the wick, pierce the mold with a wicking needle, making a hole just large enough to fit the wick snugly when threaded through. Make a collar out of cardboard to hold the lip of the mold and use a stand or vase to support it. As stearin rots rubber, the addition of Vybar is used instead to help improve the burning time and color of the wax. This candle measures 2½ inches in diameter and is 7 inches tall.

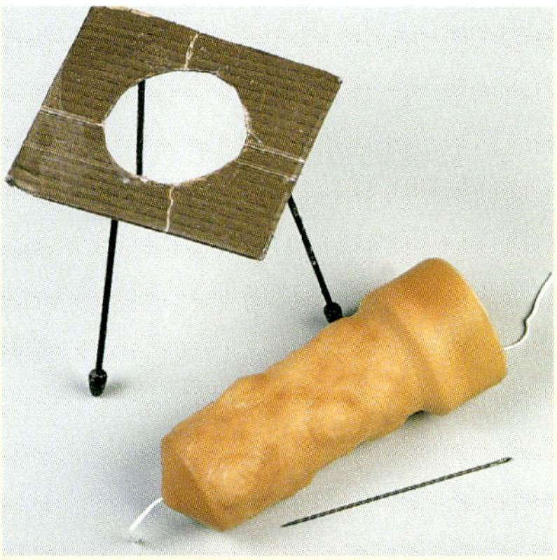

1 Make a hole in the bottom of the mold with a wicking needle and thread the wick through the mold. Tie the top end of the wick to a wicking needle resting across the mold. Make a cardboard collar to support the lip of the mold and place it on a stand or in a vase.

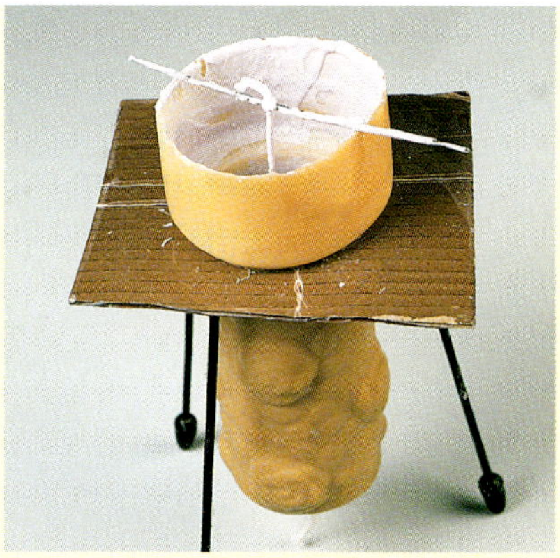

2 Melt the wax and Vybar together, adding a small amount of dye to make a pale shade. Heat it to 180°F. Pour the wax to fill the mold, then squeeze the mold to release any trapped air pockets. Leave for 5 minutes before pouring the wax back into the pan.

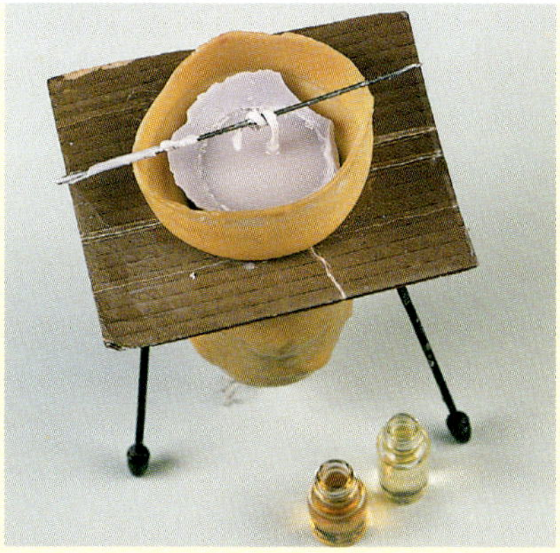

3 Reheat the wax, adding more dye to make a darker shade, and heating it to 180°F. Add the perfume and pour into the mold. Allow it to cool.

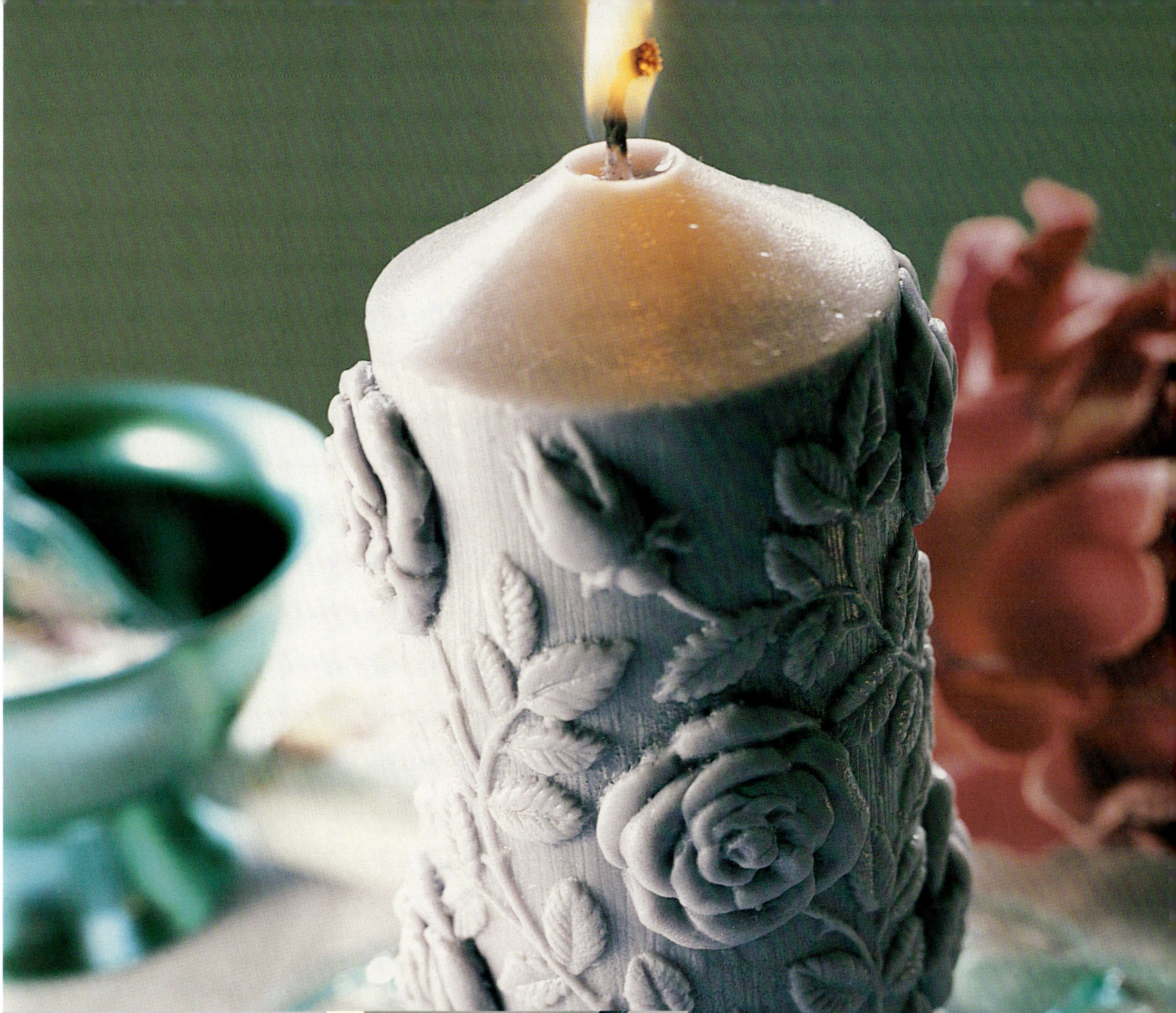

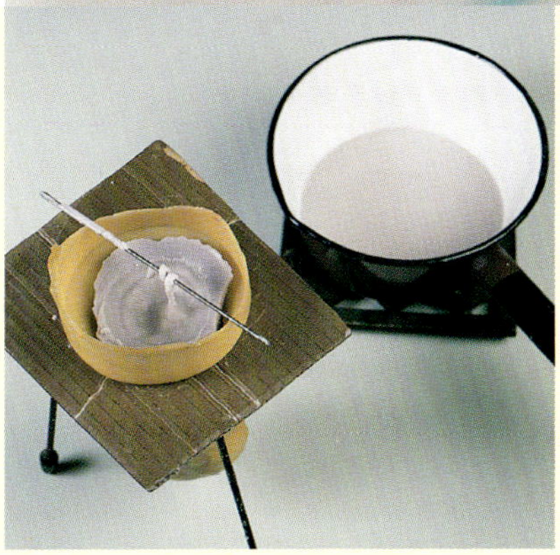

4 Reheat the wax to 180°F and fill the dip that appears around the wick. Allow the candle to completely set. Smear the mold with liquid soap and carefully peel it all the way back to remove it.

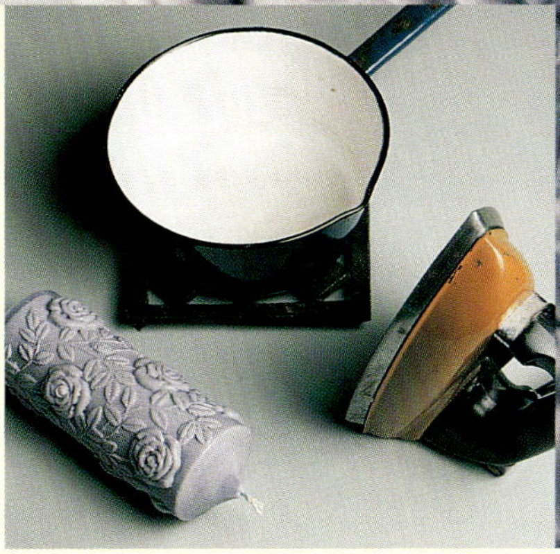

5 Trim the wick and dip in molten wax to prime it. Use a hot iron to flatten the base so the candle stands straight and steady.

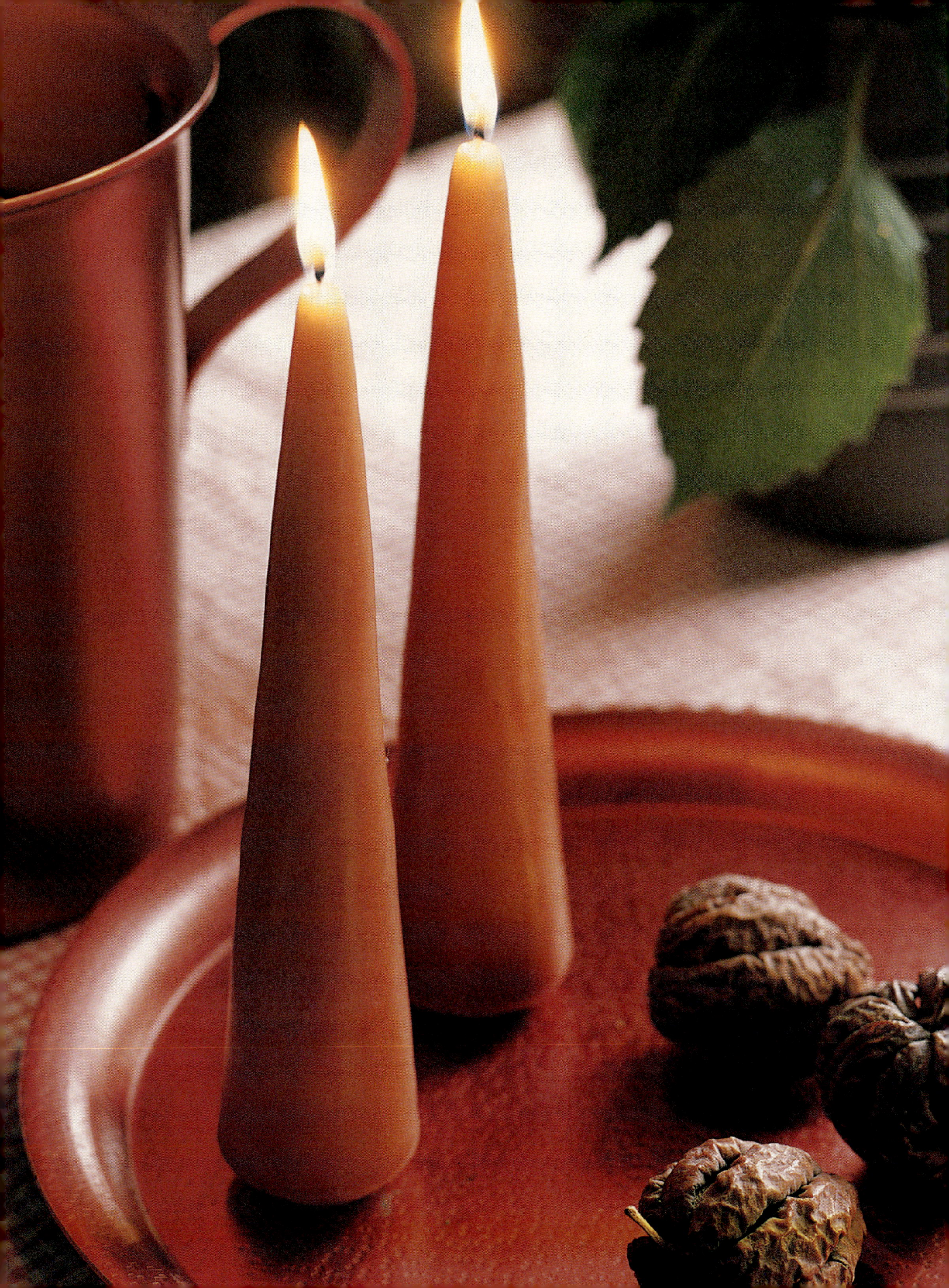

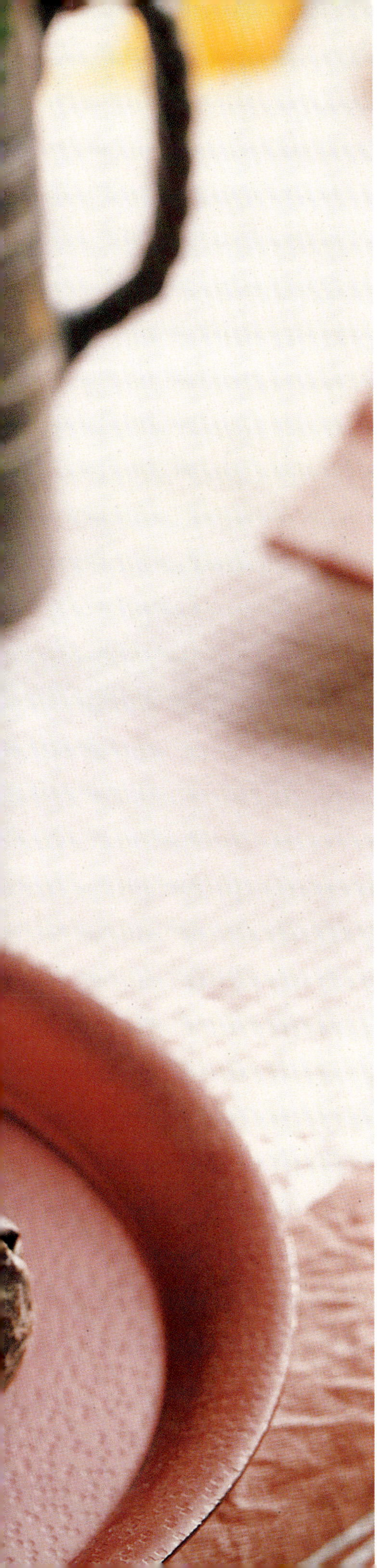

Elegant conical-shaped candles formed by dipping repeatedly in wax are scented with an exotic blend of amber and cardamom, to bring the taste of the Orient to the autumnal table.

dipped candle

Dipped candles have a wonderful handmade quality. These classic tapered candles are made in pairs by dipping a length of wick into hot wax again and again, gradually building up the shape of the candle layer upon layer. The results are fine, elegantly shaped candles with a unique quality that factory-produced candles cannot match. By perfecting the dipping technique, so that parts of the candle build up at a different rate, it is possible to form the candle into different shapes. They can be made in one solid color or simply of white wax, dipping over with a few layers of color at the end. Coated candles have a more intense color, are less likely to fade, and, when lit, glow through close to the flame in a pleasing way.

It is very satisfying to see the candles take shape before your eyes, but it does take a while for the layers to build up enough to form the finished candles. Standing over a dipping can of scented wax could become a rather tiring experience, give you a headache, or even put you off the scent for life as you continually breathe in the aroma at close quarters. For this reason, make the candle in unscented wax; when the main shape of the candle has developed, spoon a few layers of scented wax over the top, finishing with the final few dips in unscented wax. Dipping cans come in various sizes from craft suppliers, but it is possible to find an alternative that does the job just as well, such as an empty food can with clean, smooth edges. Remember that the can needs to be slightly deeper than the length of candle you wish to produce, and place the can in a pan of boiling water, similar to a double boiler, as before. Dipping cans do take a huge amount of wax, the actual quantity depending on the size of can, but as a rule allow 6½ lb. cold wax for a can 12 inches high and 5¼ inches in diameter.

you will need:

Prepared wick
Enough paraffin wax to fill a dipping can
2 tsp. wax perfume
8 oz. paraffin wax
Wax dye
⅛ oz. Vybar

MAKING THE CANDLES The candles are made in pairs. One long wick held at the center forms a candle at each end. The warm candles have a strange attraction to one another so it is important they are held apart during dipping and hung between dips so they cannot touch. Changing the dipping sequence creates variations in the final shape and can take practice. For a conical shape, the dips become shallower, gradually building up the base of the candle more than the top. The temperature of the molten wax is crucial—if too hot, the previous layer begins to melt; if too cool, bumps can appear on the candle. Adding a tiny amount of Vybar (0.2 percent) to the colored wax for the final dips improves the appearance, and a final dip at 180°F gives a smooth finish. Allow to cool for one hour before burning. These candles measure 1½ inches in diameter at the base and 8 inches high. Each takes 5 oz. wax.

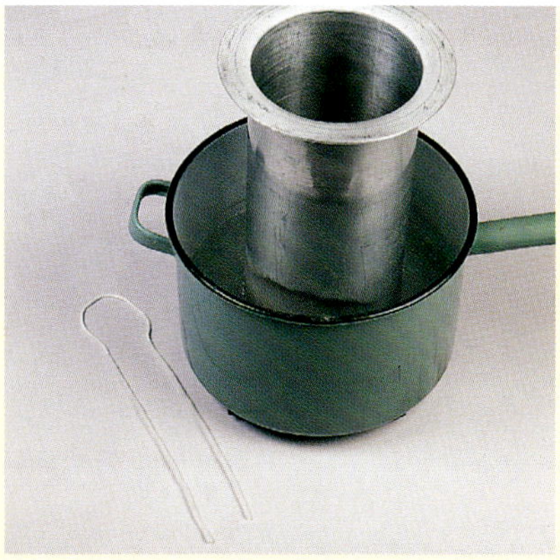

1 Melt the paraffin wax in a dipping can placed in a pan of simmering water. Heat to 160°F, then, keeping the temperature constant, hold the wick at the center and dip the ends into the wax, holding them under for 1 minute. Allow the wick to cool.

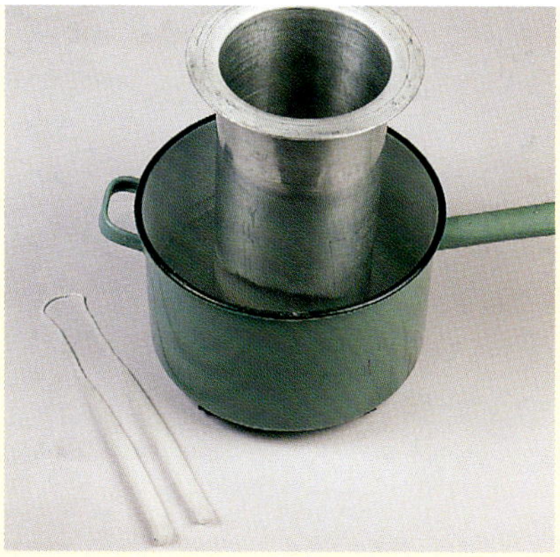

2 Begin to dip in sequence, holding the wick submerged for about 3 seconds, then allowing it to cool for 1–4 minutes, depending on the room temperature. Repeat the process until the candles begin to take form. If the surface wrinkles, they need to cool for longer between dips.

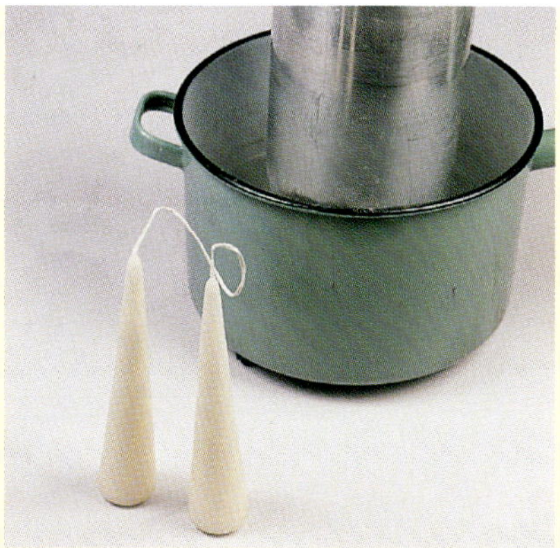

3 To form a conical shape, when the top of the candle is the required size, begin to make shallower dips, in gradations of approximately ½ inch, dipping at each level several times. In this way the candles will be dipped many more times at the base than at the top. As the candles develop, stand them on their bases to cool.

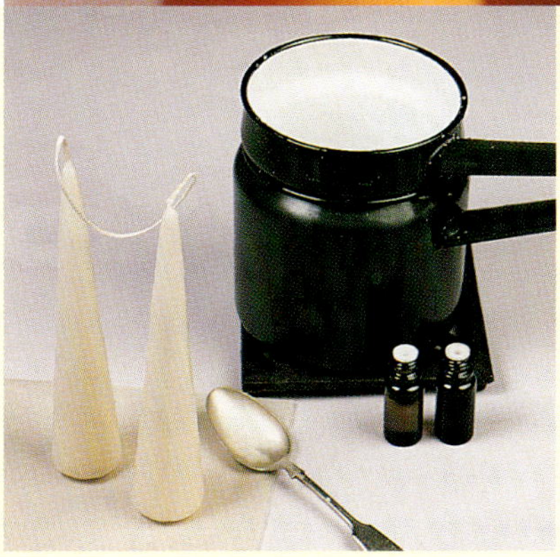

4 When the candles have reached the required thickness, melt some paraffin wax in a double boiler. Heat to 180°F and add the perfume. Stand the candles on paper to protect the table surface and spoon a few coats of the scented wax over each candle.

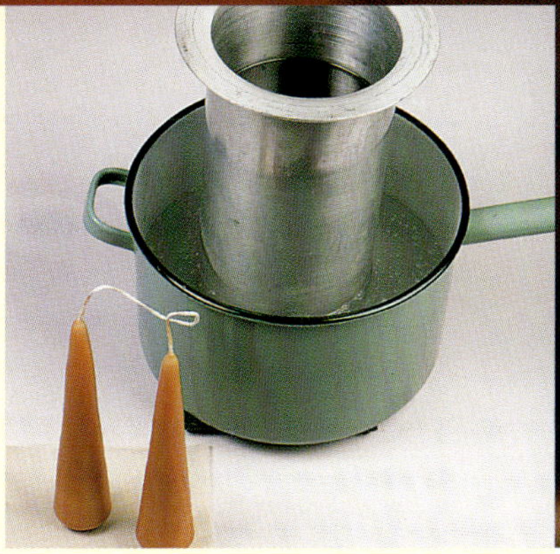

5 Heat more paraffin wax in another dipping can, add wax dye to the required shade, then add the Vybar. (If you have made all the candles you require, add the dye to the wax in the original dipping can.) Dip the candles a few times with colored wax, heating the wax to 180°F for the final, smoothing dip. Flatten each base with a hot iron and trim the wicks.

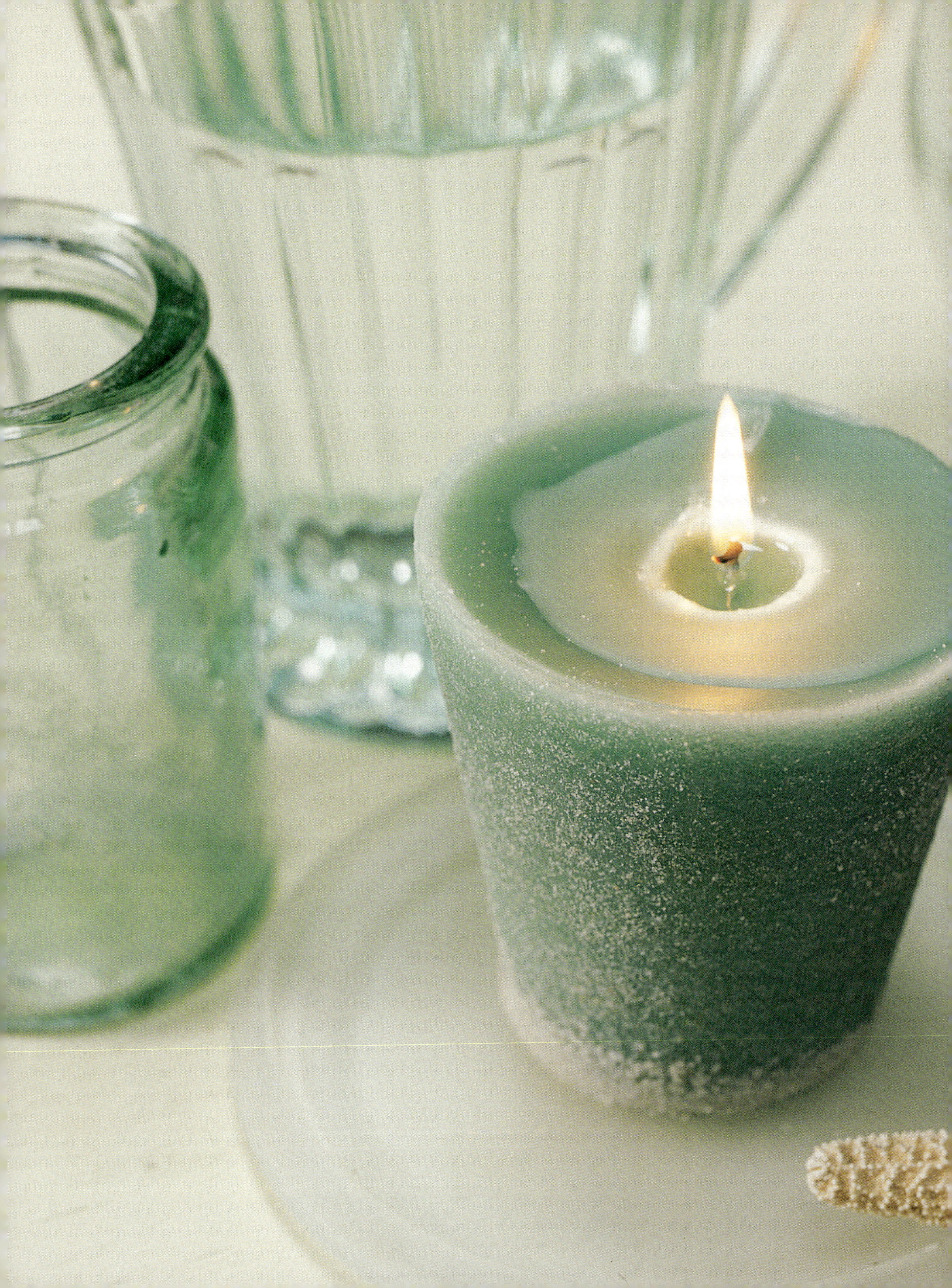

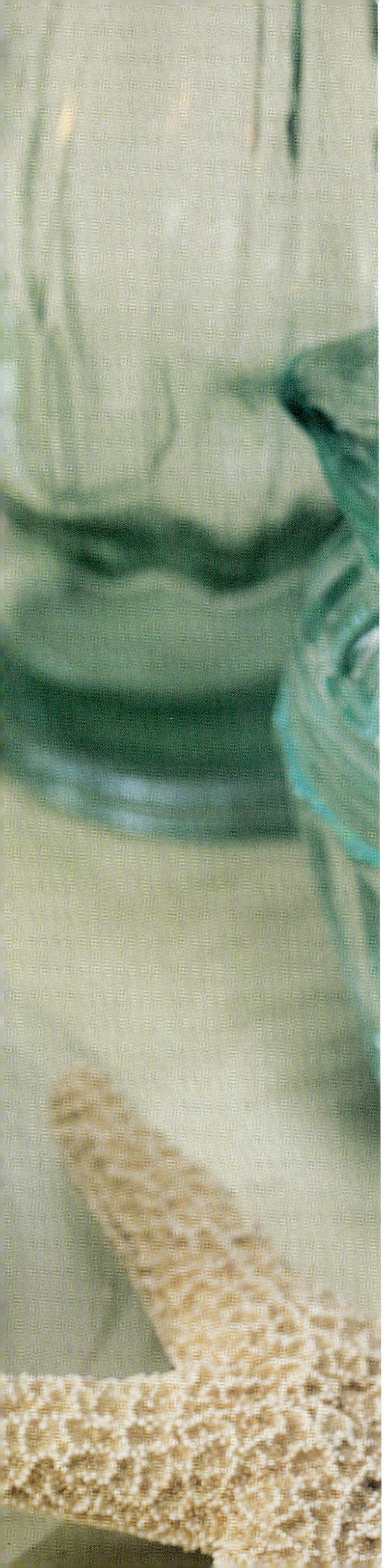

The beeswax content of this candle gives the color a luscious creamy quality that delicately complements the fine dusting of silver sand on the outside.

sand candle

Sand candles were popular in the 1960s when candle making was a fashionable pastime, and every hippie household had a crusty, rainbow-colored candle. The updated version is far more stylish and would grace any modern interior with its restrained quality. By using damp sand to make the mold, you are not limited to shapes available for buying. Simply remember that the container used to make the impression in the sand must be wider at the top than the bottom, so it pulls smoothly out of the sand. The frosted surface provides a delicate finish, so display the candles on frosted glass to accentuate this. As uplifting as breathing fresh air on an energizing walk along the beach, the light, citrus scents of mandarin and grapefruit blend effortlessly with amber, the warm and exotic scent of the Orient.

Silver sand is the finest quality and has a light color that suits this candle. The addition of beeswax to paraffin wax prolongs the candle's burning time and softens the color the dye produces. Use any proportion of cream beeswax to paraffin wax and watch how the color changes as the beeswax is added. You can vary the amount of sand that adheres to the candle by regulating the heat of the wax, but take care when adding perfume to very hot wax as the perfume can lower the flash point (the lowest temperature at which vapors ignite) and become a fire hazard.

you will need:

Straight-sided tumbler
Bucket of damp silver sand
Prepared wick
Wick sustainer
16 oz. paraffin wax and cream beeswax in total
Wax dye
1 fl. oz. wax perfume

MAKING THE CANDLE The temperature of the wax before pouring changes the look of the candle. A temperature of 200°F will give a fine dusting to the surface while at a higher temperature, up to 260°F, the wax will seep into the sand to form a thick solid coating that completely encases the sides. To heat the wax to the higher end of the scale, it may be necessary to place the pan directly on the flame as it will not be possible to attain the temperature using a double boiler. This can be a dangerous operation, so take great care. Never add perfume to wax heated to high temperatures as this increases the fire risks—scent only the wax used to fill the dips in the candle. This candle measures 3½ inches in diameter by 4 inches high.

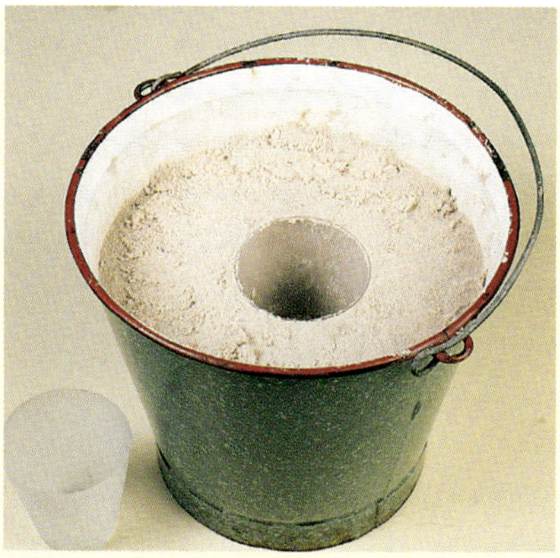

1 Choose a straight-sided tumbler for its simple lines or an oval-shaped tank vase with straight sides to make the impression in the sand for the mold. The sand needs to be damp, so combine water with dry sand, mixing it with your hands until it will hold an imprint when packed firmly.

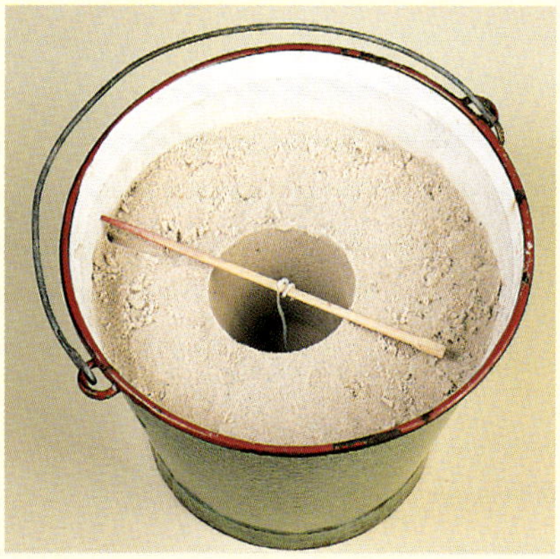

3 Attach a wick sustainer to the end of the wick, tightening the metal with pliers to secure it and place centrally in the mold. Wrap the excess wick around a wicking needle or stick resting across the top of the hole.

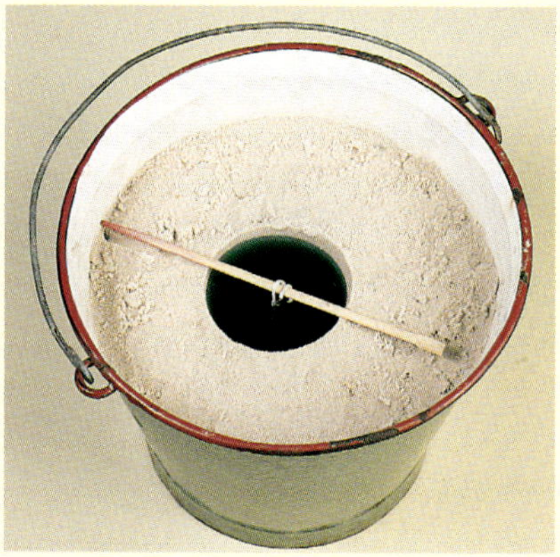

4 Heat the wax and beeswax, then add dye to the required shade. When it reaches 200°F, add the perfume, then with a steady hand pour the wax carefully into the mold, trying to avoid any splashes. Allow it to set.

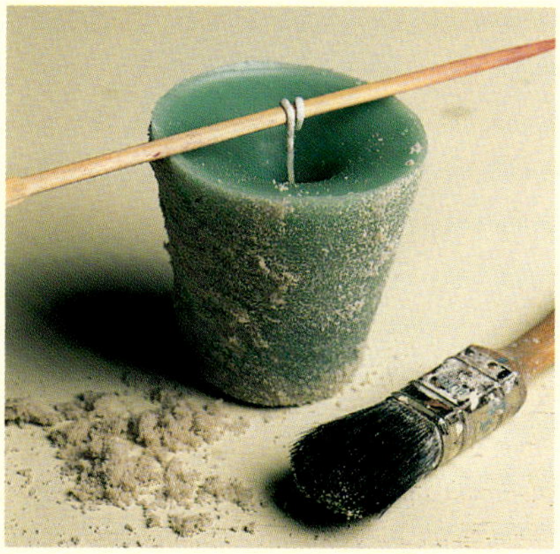

5 When the wax is completely set, remove the candle from the mold and brush away the excess sand from the surface. Run a hot iron over the base if necessary so the candle sits straight when burning.

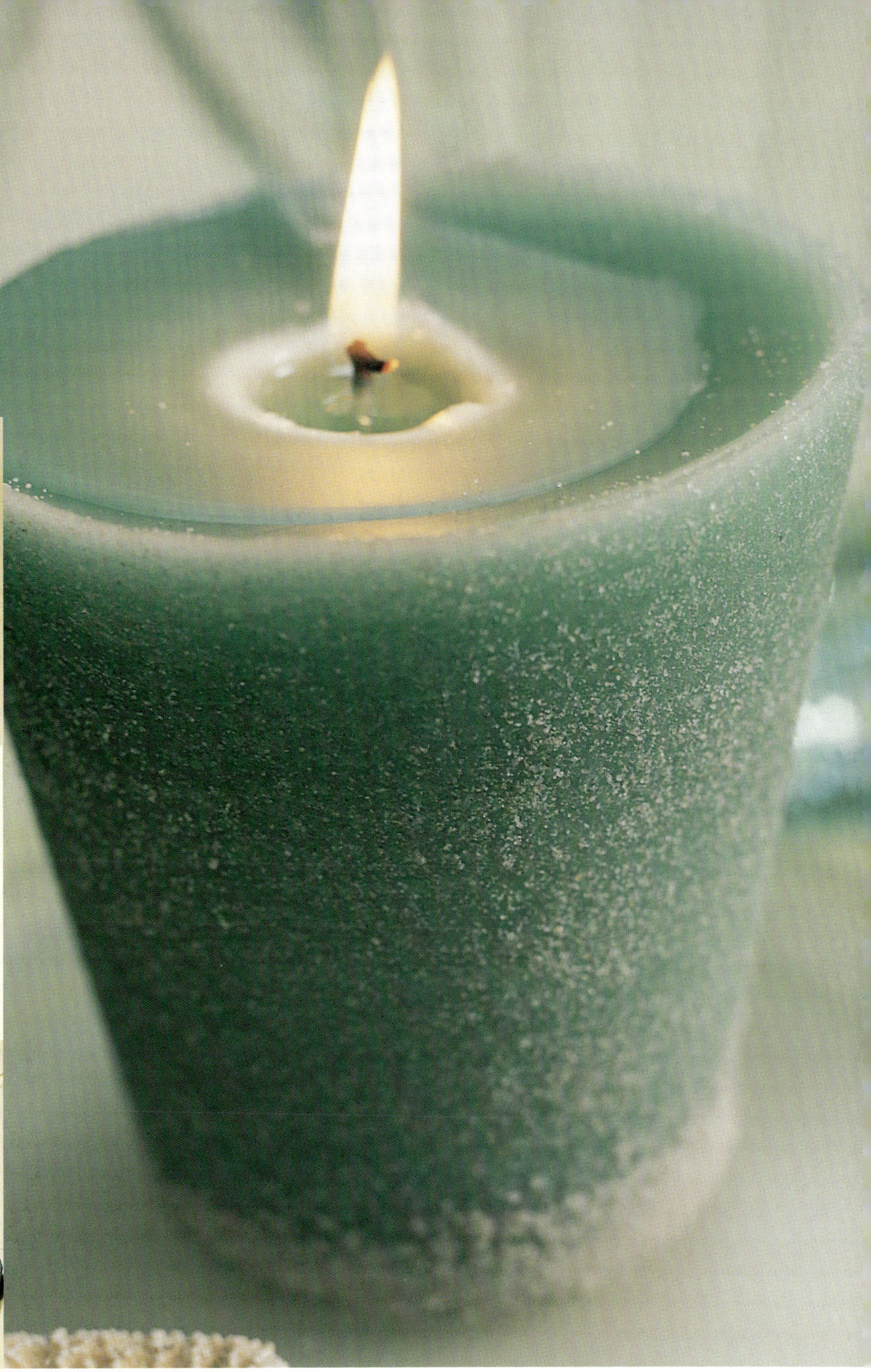

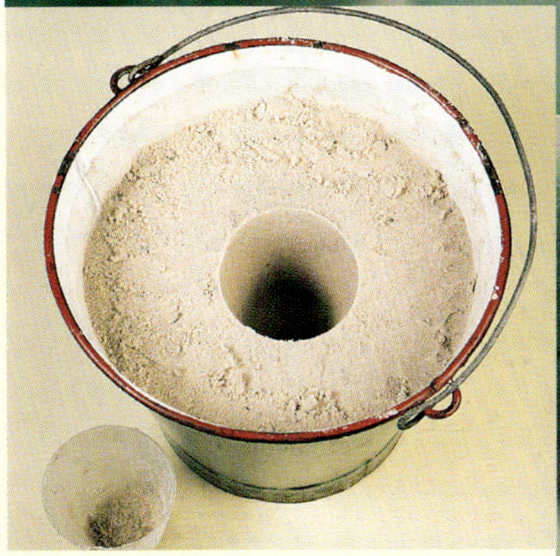

2 To form the mold, push the tumbler into the center of the damp sand in the bucket and pack the sand really firmly around it. Carefully lift the tumbler away to leave a perfect, smooth impression of the glass in the sand.

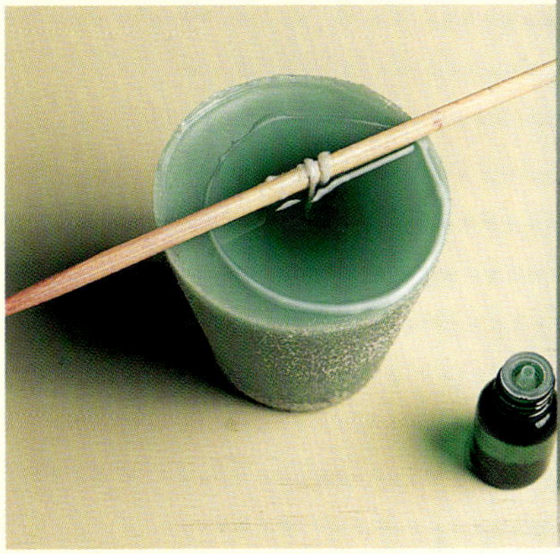

6 Reheat some wax and fill the dip in the top of the candle, taking care that molten wax doesn't run over the rim. Allow to set, then remove the wicking needle and trim the wick.

This impressive bowl candle looks more technically challenging to make than it actually is. It is in fact a container candle with the outer bowl made of wax to provide the container. This candle creates a vibrancy as it burns; the light from the flame radiates through the wax walls of the bowl for a stunning effect. Wax bowls can be displayed as part of a table setting for a special dinner party, filled with fruit and flowers. As they are watertight, they can be used with floating candles or simply styled with real blossoms bobbing on water. This richly colored candle is scented with the warm and exotic citrus scent of orange, with a sprinkling of spicy nutmeg to bring inspiration and cheer to a crisp fall evening.

bowl candle

you will need:

3½ pint glass bowl
1 oz. stearin
Wax dye
3 lb. paraffin wax
Prepared medium container wick
Wick sustainer
Approximately 1 tsp. essential oil or candle perfume

MAKING THE CANDLE Using a level, make sure your work surface is perfectly flat, so the finished candle will have a symmetrical shape. You need enough wax to completely fill the mold as the molten wax is poured in right up to the rim, then left to set for the bowl sides to form. The wax inside the bowl is then poured back into the pan and used to make the filling for the candle. Pouring the wax into the mold at a lower temperature will give the wax an interesting frosted surface texture. There is no need to scent the wax for the bowl itself—just fragrance the candle filling. This bowl measures 7 inches diameter across the rim and 4 inches deep.

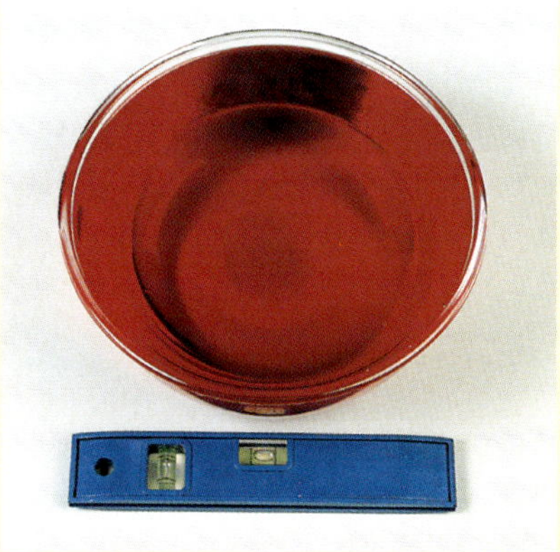

1 Melt the stearin and dye together and add the paraffin wax. Heat to 160°F. Check that the tabletop is flat using a level. Fill the bowl with wax and allow it to cool.

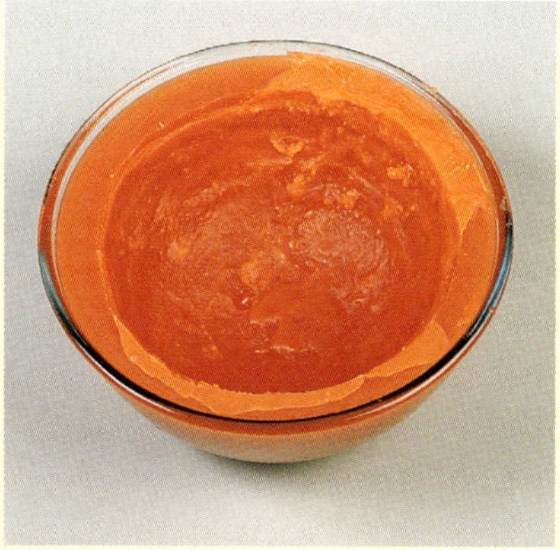

2 When the wax has begun to set and the bowl sides are approximately ½ inch thick, break the wax that has set on the surface of the candle and pour out the molten wax from the center to form a bowl. Use a spoon to even out the surface.

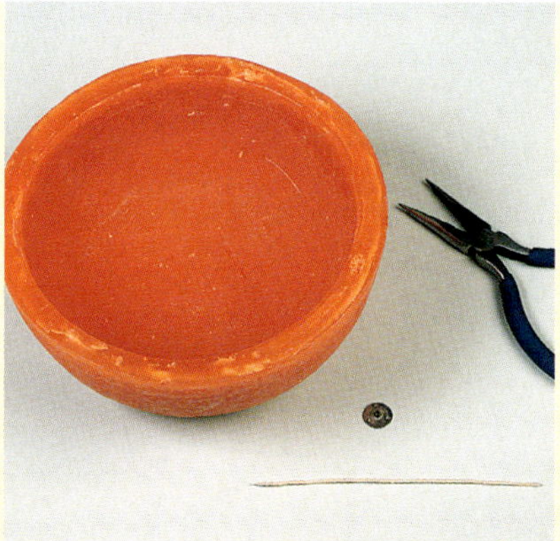

3 Allow the bowl to cool and use a hot iron to flatten and smooth the wax around the rim. Attach a wick sustainer to the end of the primed wick by squeezing the metal tightly closed with pliers around the wick.

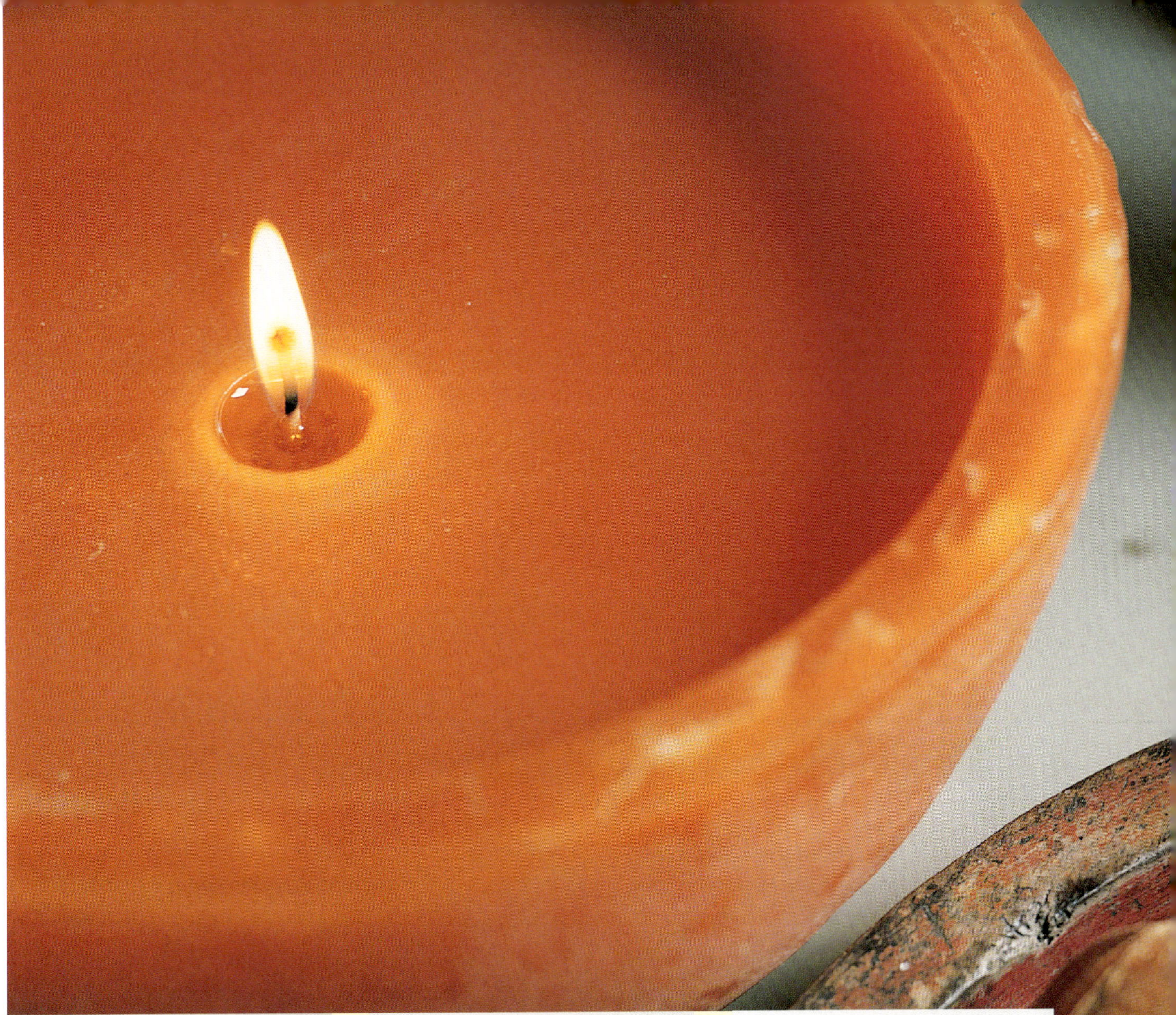

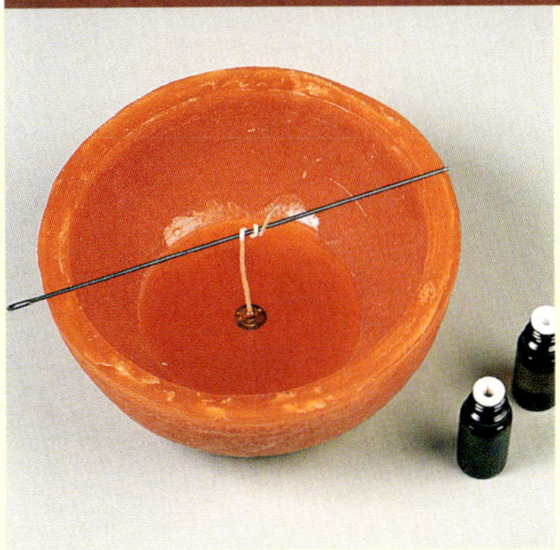

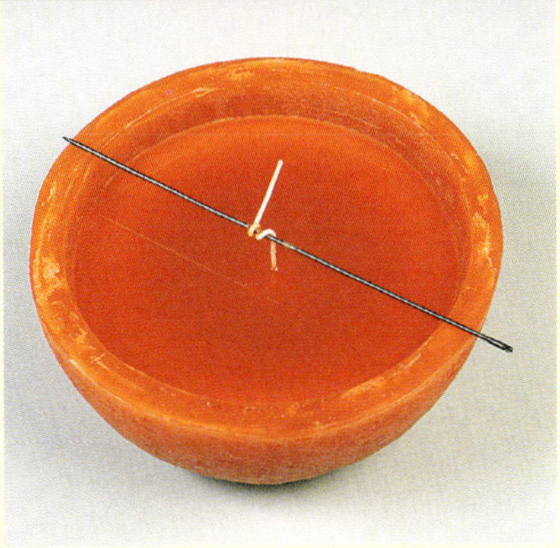

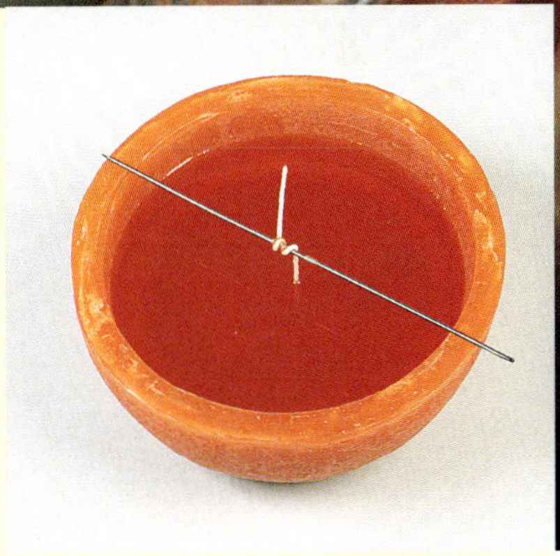

4 Place the wick centrally inside the bowl with the sustainer sitting on the bottom of the bowl. Wrap the end of the wick around a wicking needle resting across the bowl. Reheat the wax and pour a small amount into the bowl. Allow to set.

5 Reheat the wax to 160°F and add the perfume. Pour it into the bowl, filling it to within 1 inch of the rim. Allow to cool.

6 Reheat the wax and fill any dips that have appeared on the surface around the wick. Allow to set. Remove the wicking needle and trim the wick.

Tall, elegant dipped candles radiate warmth and cheerfulness in these rich oranges, russets, and reds of fall leaves.

FALL COLORS

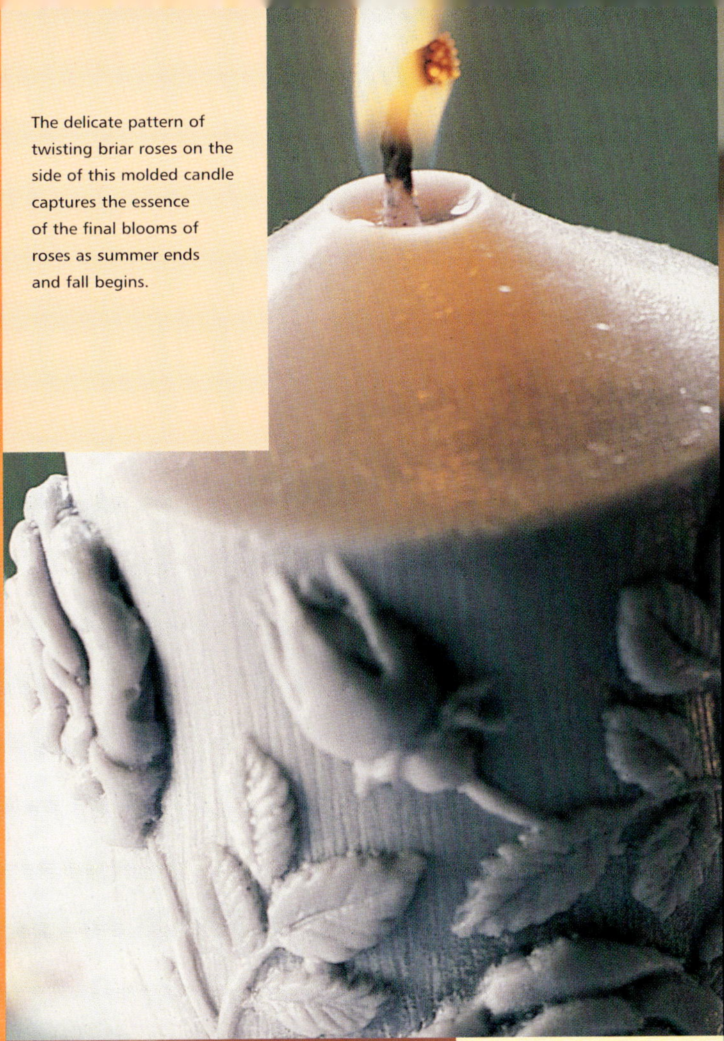

The delicate pattern of twisting briar roses on the side of this molded candle captures the essence of the final blooms of roses as summer ends and fall begins.

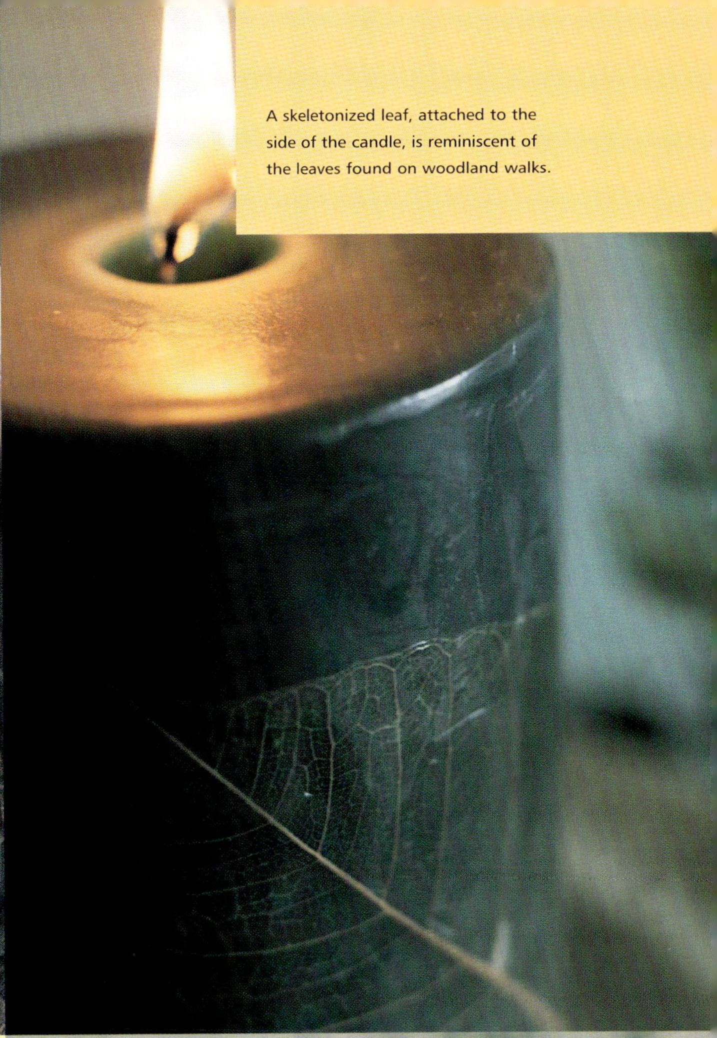

A skeletonized leaf, attached to the side of the candle, is reminiscent of the leaves found on woodland walks.

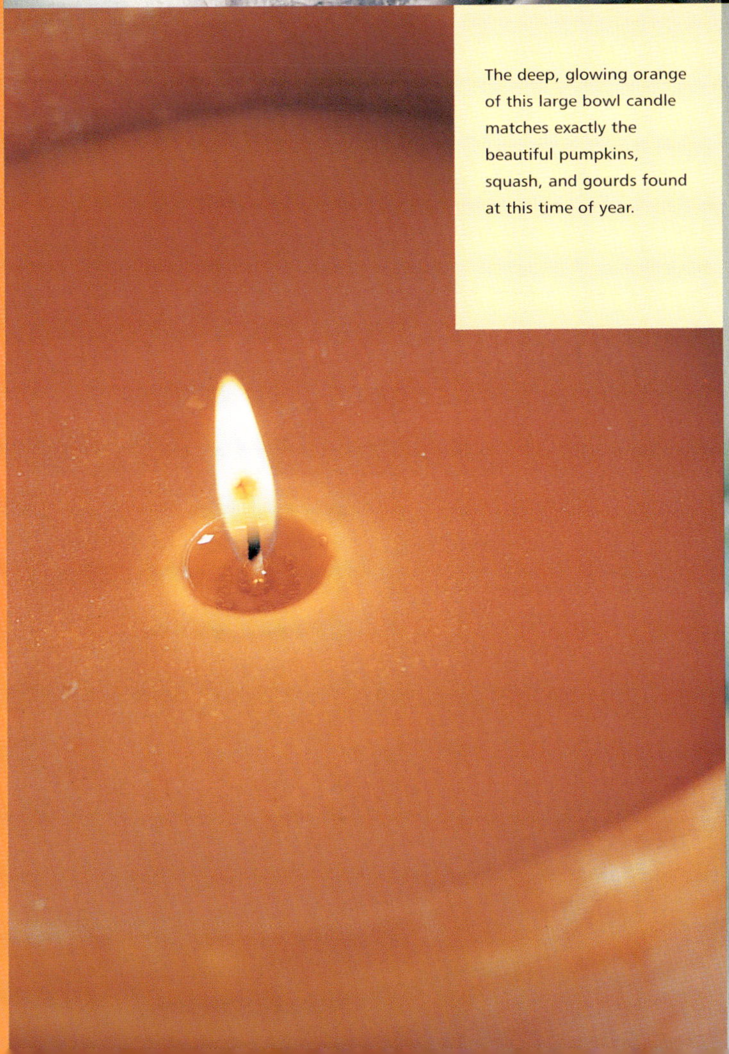

The deep, glowing orange of this large bowl candle matches exactly the beautiful pumpkins, squash, and gourds found at this time of year.

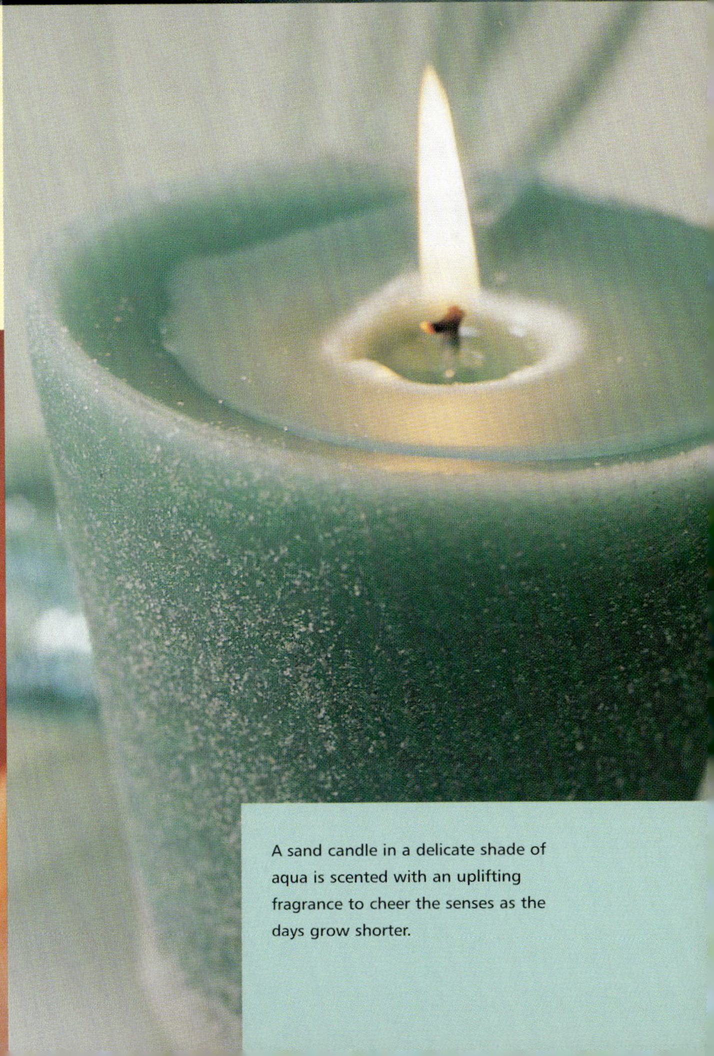

A sand candle in a delicate shade of aqua is scented with an uplifting fragrance to cheer the senses as the days grow shorter.

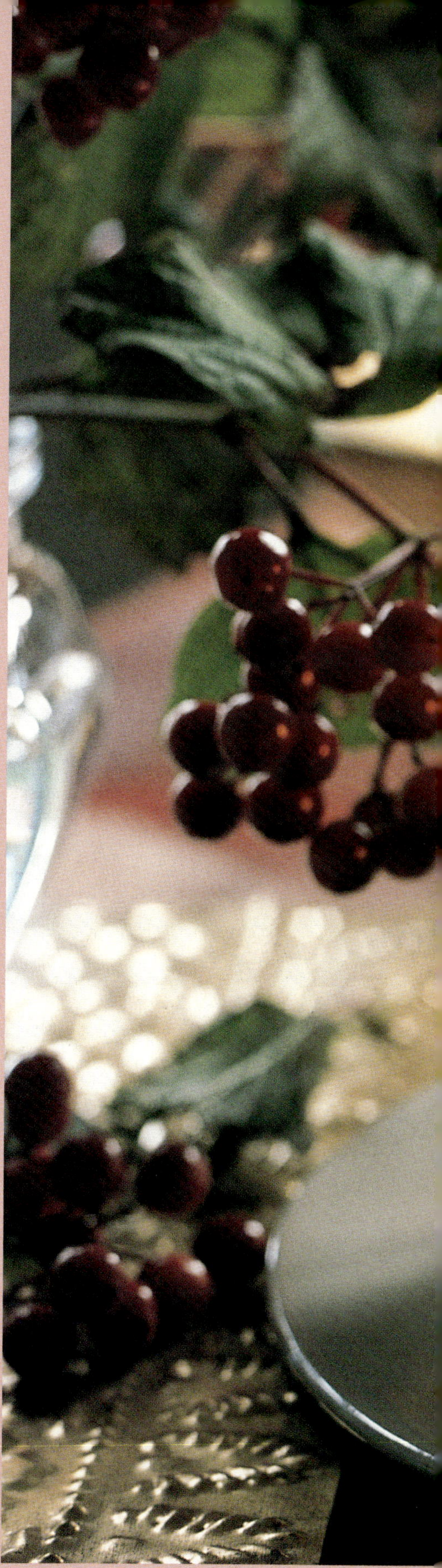

ESSENCE OF winter

With Christmas and New Year celebrations to look forward to, the cold, dark days of winter are scarcely in evidence as the home becomes a hive of activity. Candlelight adds a sparkle to the proceedings and is an essential element for gatherings and parties. The flickering flames of an open fire and a mantel decorated with candlelight complement each other perfectly, bringing comfort and warmth to the house. It is a time for family get-togethers, customs, and rituals. Candles in rich colors and scented with the fragrances of the season's fruits and spices are a vital part of decorating schemes for high feasts and festivals, and to mark the beginning of a new year.

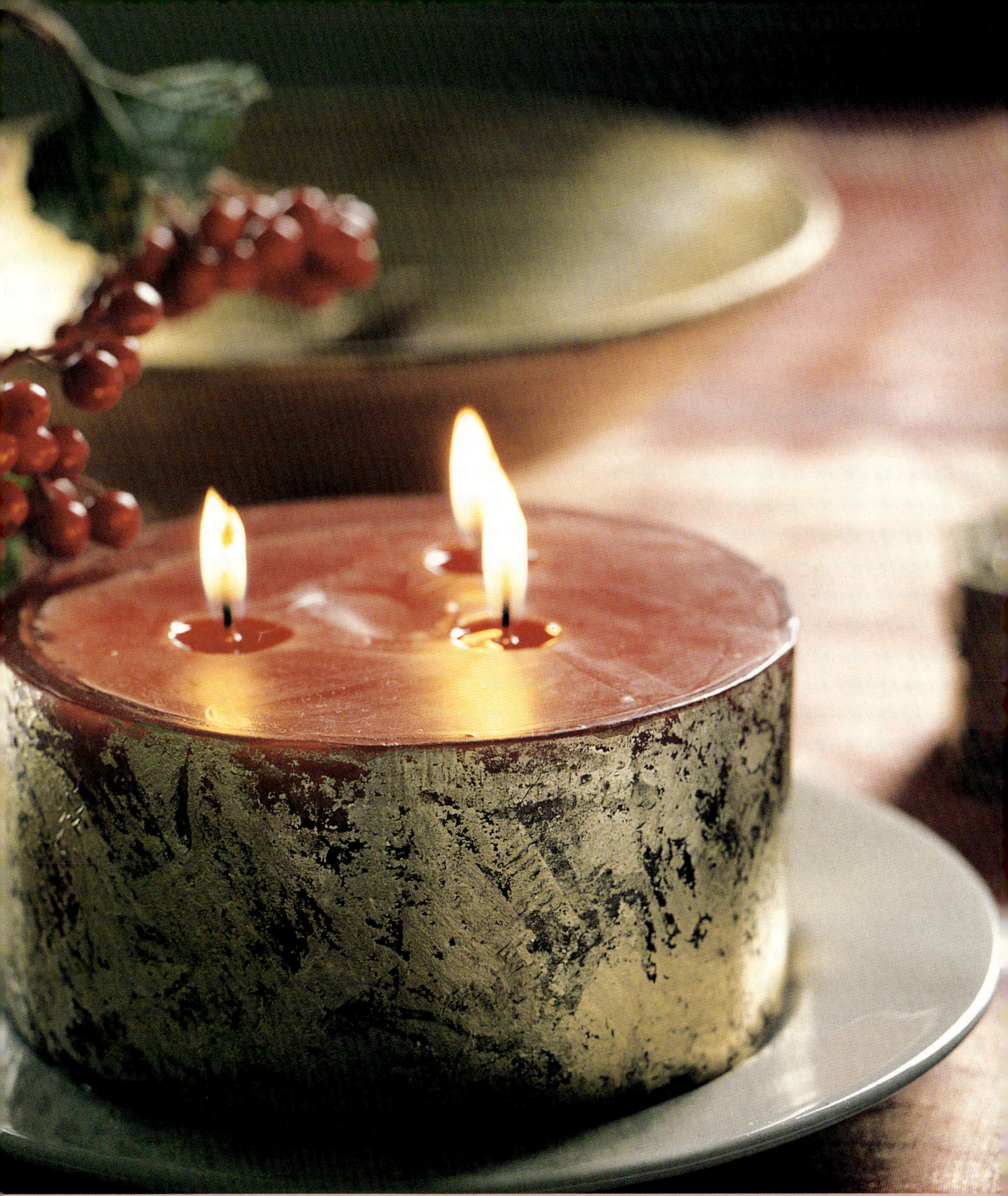

Gilded surfaces glimmer when bathed in candlelight in a truly luxurious way. A pillar candle in rich, festive red is scented with frankincense and myrrh, a seasonal blend that is both soothing and spiritual.

Cube candles have a classic look that fits in anywhere, but especially in modern settings. They are easy to make by recycling old milk cartons to use as molds. Craft stores now sell wax dyes in shades that exactly mimic the colors of white, milk, and plain chocolate, which takes the guesswork out of mixing the colors yourself. The results give an authentic look, just like the real thing. Choose the obvious combination of scents to complement these candles by using the warm, comforting fragrances of chocolate and vanilla. Pouring the wax into the mold at a lower temperature will give an interesting frosted texture to the surfaces.

cube candle

you will need:

Empty milk carton
Prepared wick
Wick sustainer
2 oz. stearin
Wax dye
9 oz. paraffin wax
Approximately 3 tsp. candle perfume

MAKING THE CANDLE Empty milk cartons constructed from waxed cardboard make ideal molds for cube and square column candles. Wash and dry an empty carton thoroughly and cut off the folded top part before you begin. It is well worth reinforcing the outside of the carton with pieces of cardboard so the sides of the candle will stay flat and not bow outward when filled with hot wax. To make a perfect cube, measure the base and then mark the insides of the mold with a permanent marker so you know how high to fill it. When the candle is complete, just tear the carton away. This candle measures 2¾ by 2¾ inches.

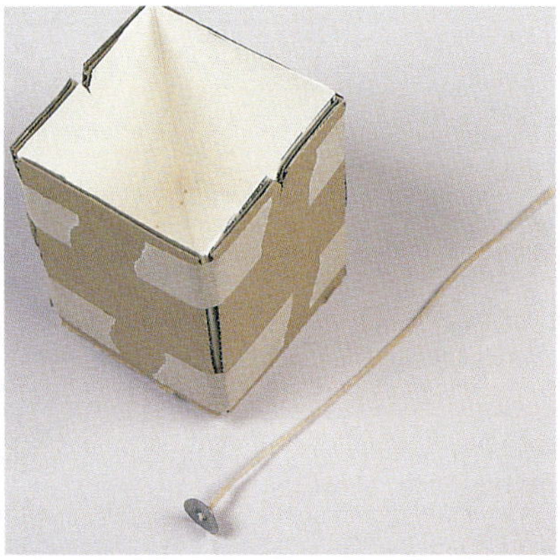

1 Reinforce the sides of the mold with pieces of cardboard taped to the outside of the carton with masking tape. Cut away two small "V"shapes at the center of two facing sides. Attach the wick sustainer to one end of the wick, tightening the metal with pliers.

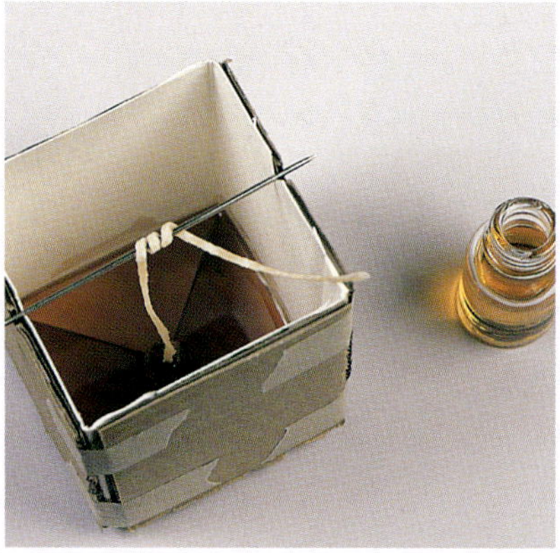

2 Place the wick centrally in the mold with the sustainer resting on the base. Wind the excess wick around a wicking needle resting in the cut-out "V" shapes. Melt the stearin and dye, then add the wax and heat to 150°F. Add the perfume and pour a thin layer into the mold. Allow to cool slightly.

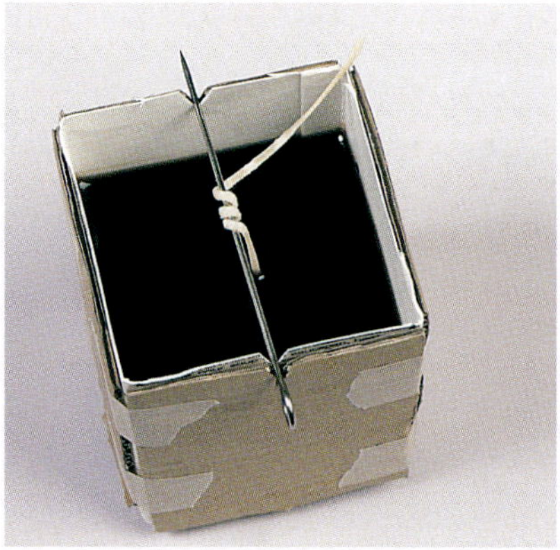

3 Reheat the wax to 150°F, as before, and pour into the mold to the same depth as the width of the mold to form a cube. Allow the candle to cool.

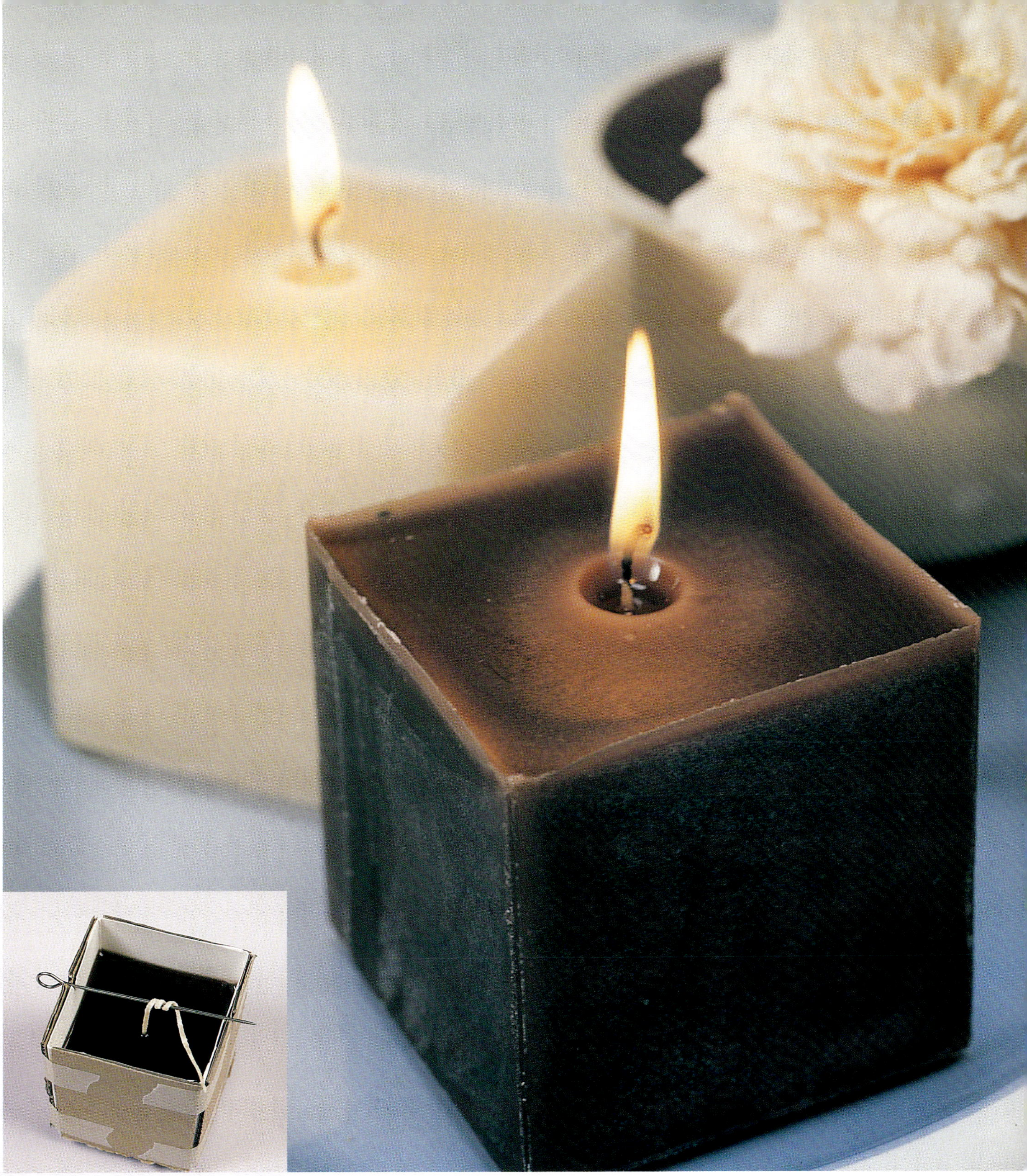

4 Reheat the wax again and fill the dip that forms on the surface around the wick as the candle sets and shrinks. Allow to cool completely, then tear away the carton. Trim the wick.

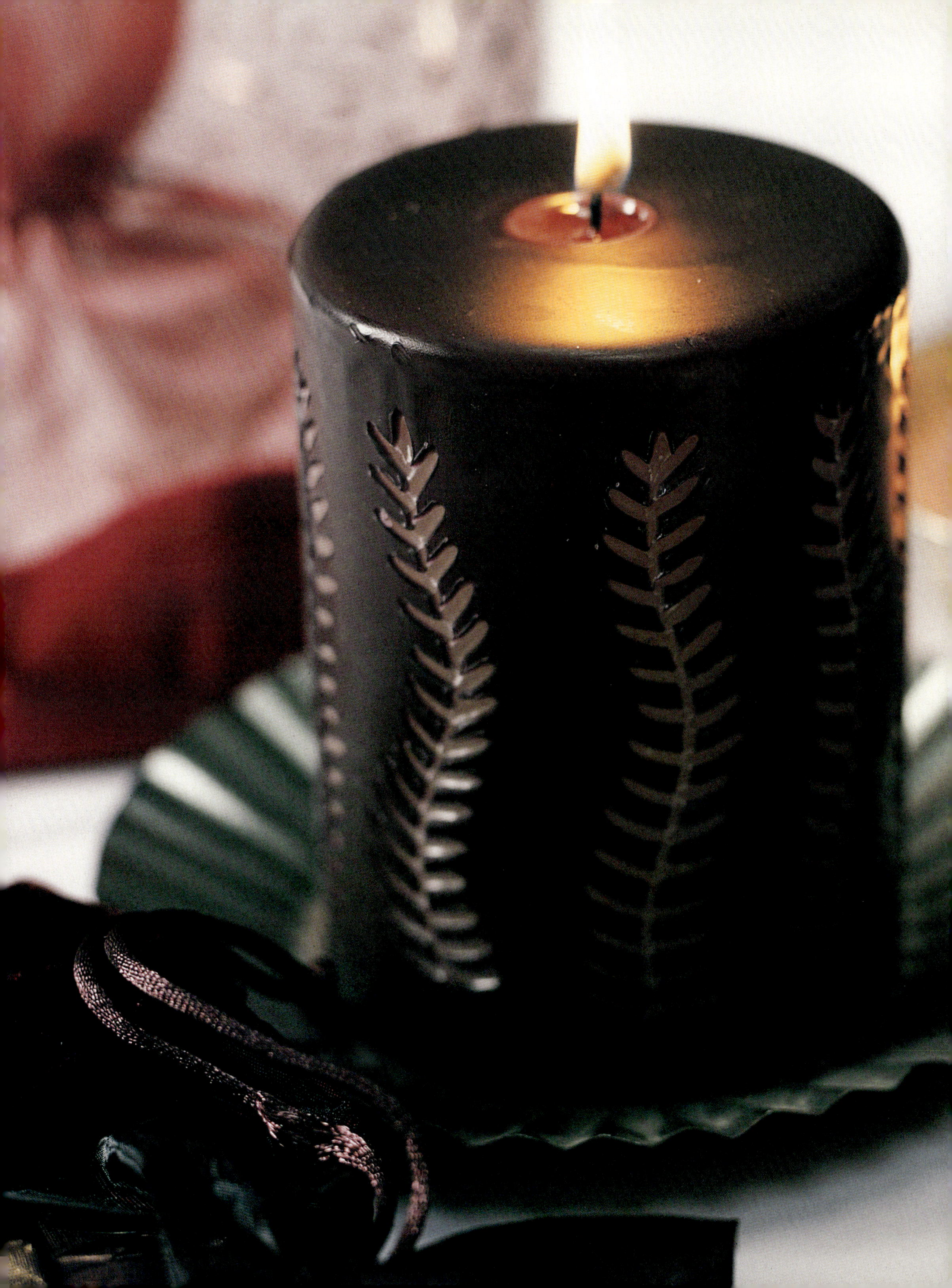

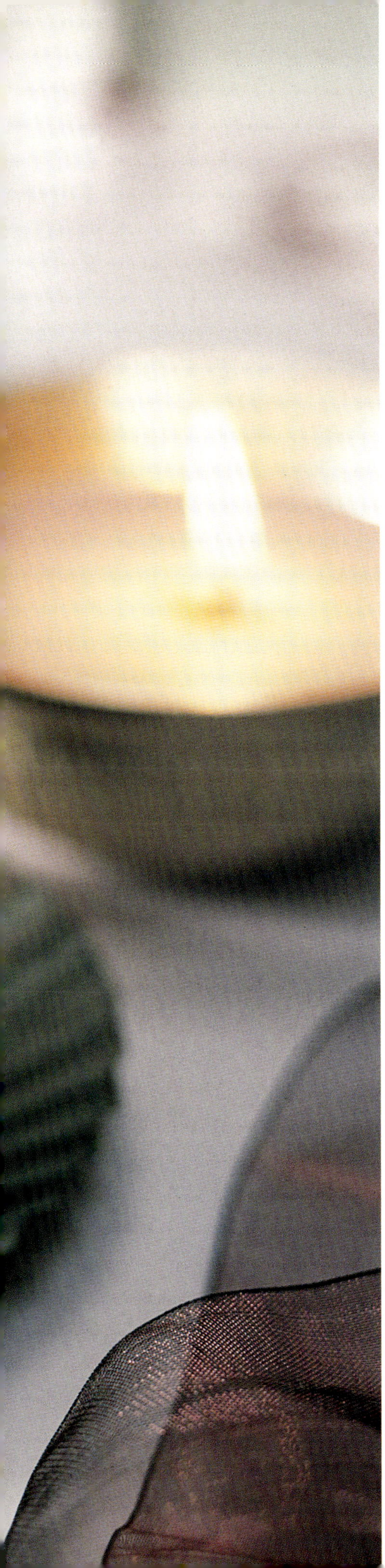

Carving patterns in the wax to uncover the paler color beneath gives a simple but luxurious effect. As the candle gradually burns, the glow illuminates the carved decoration from the inside.

carved candle

Carved candles have a wonderful three-dimensional quality and, as the wax burns down, the light from the flame glows through the carved pattern. Candles for carving need to be specially prepared to make them workable. Here, a pale cream pillar candle is dipped in a deeper color using dip-and-carve wax, which is more flexible than ordinary paraffin wax. By using a rich, dark eggplant color for the top layer, the finished candle looks particularly effective with the top layer cut away to reveal the cream wax beneath. It is worth dipping a spare candle so you can practice carving patterns to perfect the technique. Inspired by nature, a pattern of wavy lines decorates the candle and look like a stylized version of the veins of leaves.

For this project, you can dip a good-quality, cream church candle rather than making the candle from scratch if you wish, but for the best results, make your own special scented candle. Coating the candle with a few layers of a darker colored wax helps to provide a good contrast when the carved pattern is applied. Practice making the pattern using a sharp "V"-shaped lino-cutting blade and brush away any fragments of wax that stick to the carving with a small paintbrush. Mark faint guidelines on the candle's surface using a sharp pencil first, in order to position the pattern evenly over the candle. The sweet and exotic blend of tuberose and sandalwood provides a luxurious and heady fragrance and complements the opulence of this candle.

you will need:

Prepared wick
Pillar candle mold
Mold seal
4½ oz. stearin
Wax dye
1 lb. paraffin wax beads
1 fl. oz. essential oil or wax perfume
Enough dip-and-carve wax to fill a dipping can
Lino-cutting tool

MAKING THE CANDLE Fill the dipping can with enough wax so the candle becomes completely submerged when dipped in the can. Heat the wax to 180°F and, holding the candle by the wick, dip into the wax for about three seconds, allowing it to cool for a minute or two between dips. The wax should be dyed to such an intensity that a few dips will produce the required shade on the candle. The outer dipped layer needs to be as thin as possible to make carving easier. This cylinder mold measures 3¼ inches in diameter and 5 inches high.

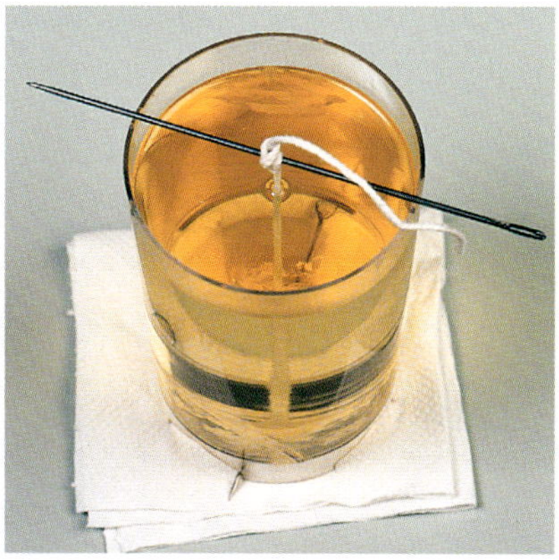

1 Thread the wick through the mold and secure it underneath with mold seal so the mold is watertight. Wrap the other end of the wick around a wicking needle resting across the rim. Melt the stearin and wax dye together, then add the paraffin wax. Heat to 200°F, add the perfume, then pour into the mold.

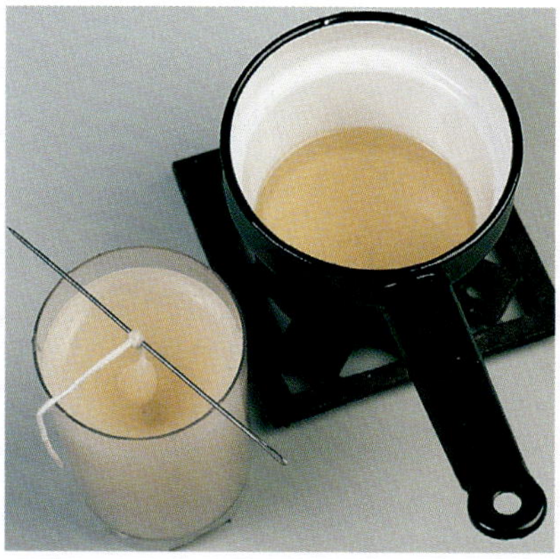

2 Allow the candle to cool in a water bath, then reheat the wax and fill the dip around the wick, taking care that no wax runs over the side between the mold and the candle. Allow to cool completely, then remove from the mold.

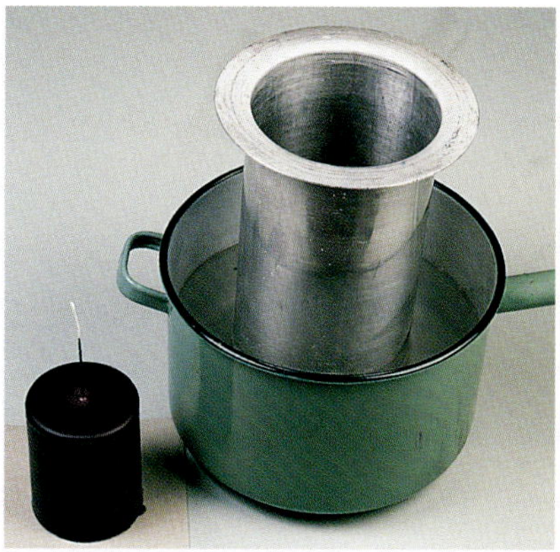

3 Place a dipping can in a pan of simmering water. Melt enough dip-and-carve wax in the can to submerge the candle when dipped. Add the dye to the wax and heat to 180°F. Holding the candle by the wick, dip it several times in the wax, allowing a few minutes between dips.

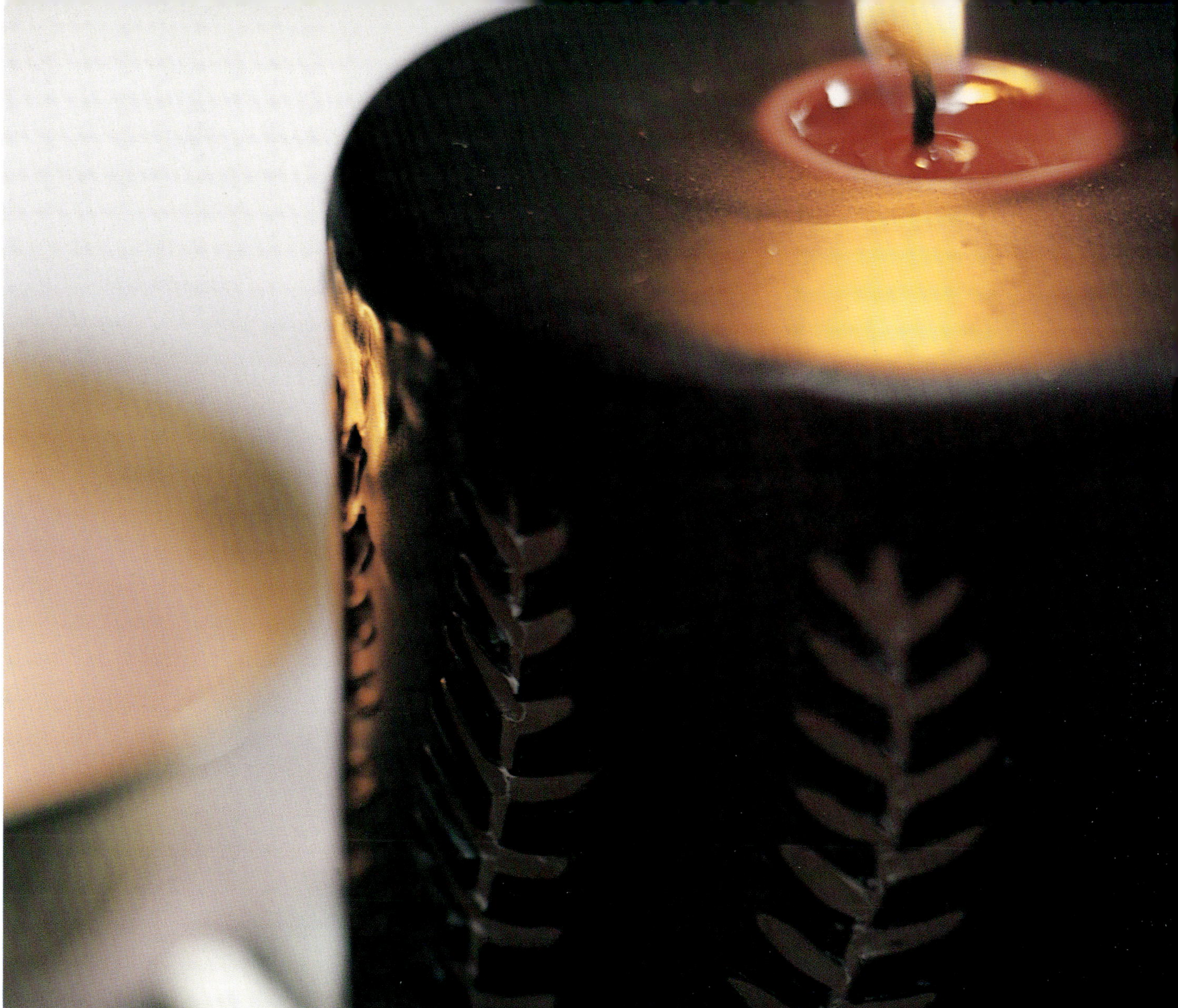

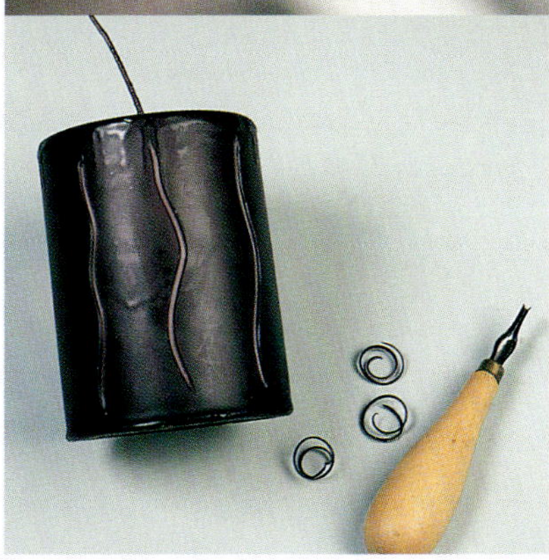

4 Using a pencil, lightly mark equidistant wavy lines around the candle. Using a lino-cutting tool, gouge out the lines cleanly with the sharp "V"-shaped blade to reveal the cream-colored candle underneath.

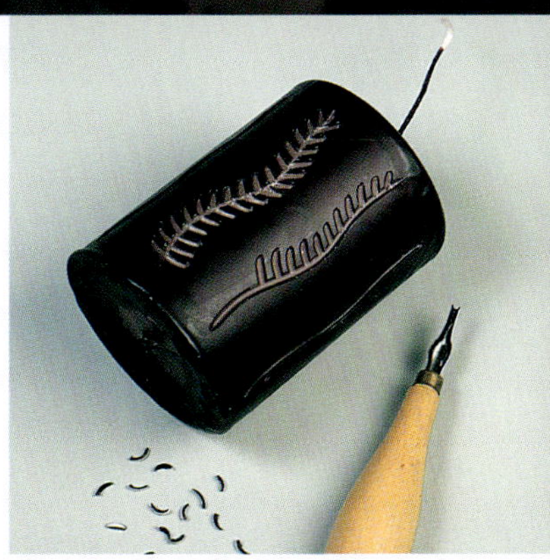

5 Working from the outside in toward the central wavy line, use the lino-cutting tool to make short marks like leaf veins so the cream candle beneath shows through. Complete the carving all the way around. Trim the wick.

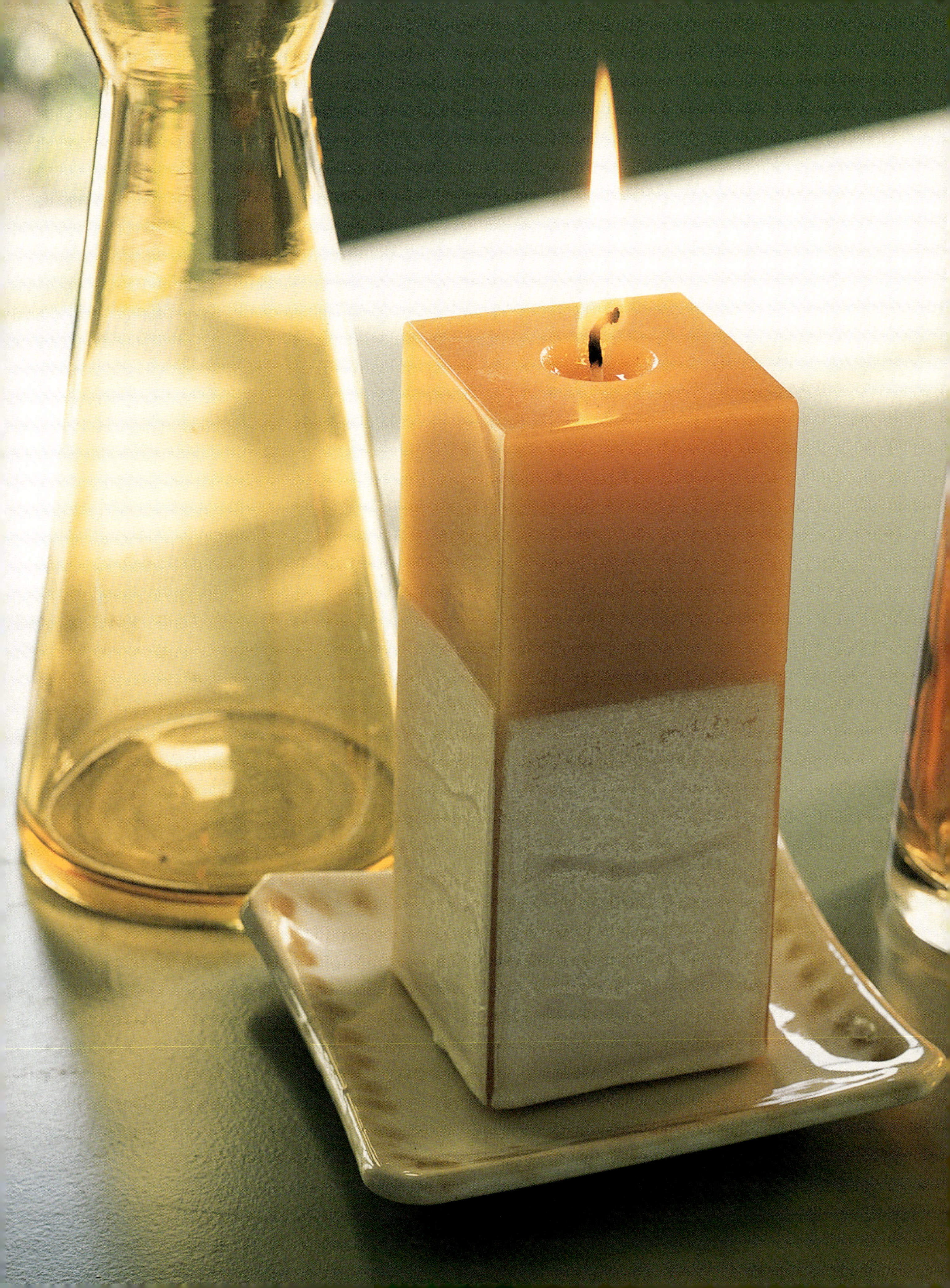

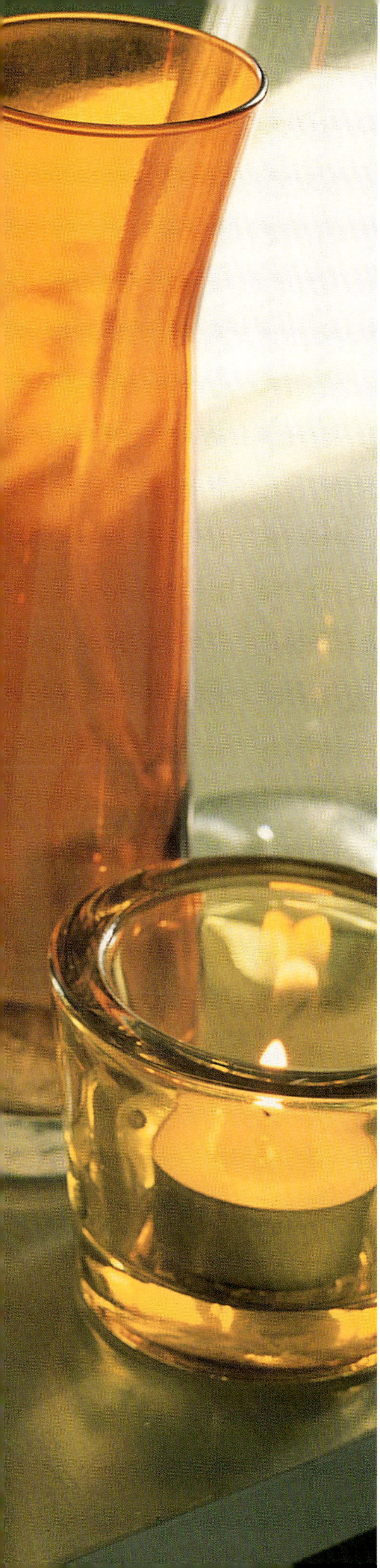

A modern pillar candle fragranced with the soothing scents of amber and oakmoss is displayed on a square ceramic dish set among colored glassware for a mellow mood.

molded candle

The clean lines of this square candle have a contemporary feel suited for a modern interior. The candle's appearance is strong enough on its own, or you could make several candles, each one dipped to a different level and display them together. This geometric design device creates blocks of contrasting color and texture simply by dipping the candle in a crystalline solution. The crystalline solution is pale and creamy with an interesting mottled texture that develops as the solution cools. The optimistic, uplifting shades of amber reflect the gold and opulence of the season, as well as echoing the warming scents of amber and oakmoss that fragrance the candle. Use rectangular dishes and colored glassware in interesting angular shapes to enhance the straight lines of the candle.

Using this crystalline dip technique creates a solid block of contrasting color and texture on the candle. The proportion of the paler dipped area to plain wax can be varied. Curved surfaces on round pillar candles look particularly good when dipped to the halfway mark or when the bottom two-thirds of the candle are enveloped in the creamy crystalline solution, giving a bold and modern effect. The dip needs to contrast with the candle, but looks best if it is a paler shade of the candle color. Use wax pigment sparingly rather than wax dye to give a hint of color to the dip. Just adding a minute amount of brown or yellow will give a pale cream color similar to the one shown. An unusual blend of oakmoss and amber is used to fragrance the candle. Oakmoss has been used as a perfume ingredient for thousands of years and imparts a faint, honeyed scent of newly mown hay.

you will need:

- Prepared wick
- Square pillar mold
- Mold seal
- 3 oz. stearin
- Wax dye
- 1 lb. paraffin wax
- Approximately 1 fl. oz. essential oil or wax perfume
- Crystalline dip
- Wax pigment

MAKING THE CANDLE The crystalline dip is very easy to handle and comes in granule form, similar to wax, which you simply melt in a pan. The crystalline dip should fill the pan when melted to the level you wish the candle to be covered to; remember some liquid will be displaced as the candle is lowered into the solution. Place the pan on a level surface so the candle sits on the base of the pan during the dipping process and the dip forms a definite edge. After dipping, place the candle on the work surface so the base stays flat and level as it cools. As the dip sets on the candle, the mottled texture appears. Allow it to cool slowly for the best results, as the longer it takes to cool, the better the effect will be. This mold measures 2½ inches square and 6 inches high.

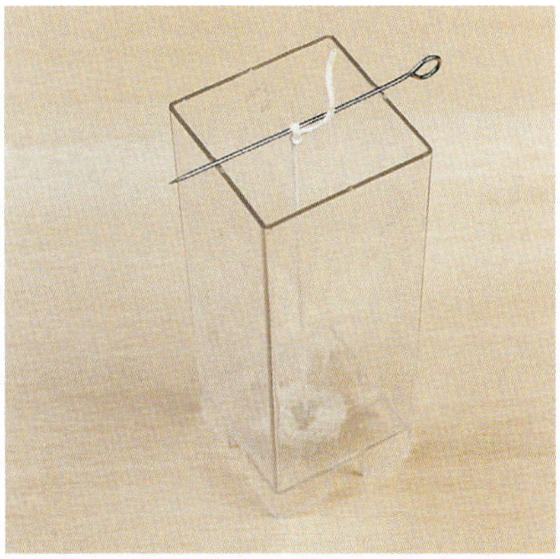

1 Thread the wick through the base of the mold and use mold seal to make it watertight. Tie the other end of the wick to a wicking needle resting across the rim of the mold.

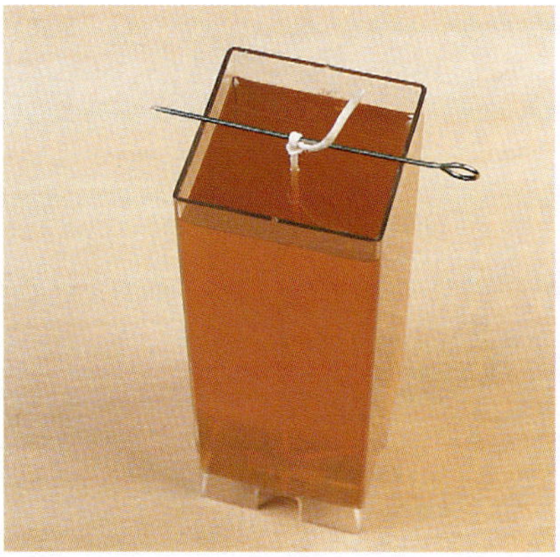

2 Heat the stearin and dye together, then add the paraffin wax. Heat the mixture to 200°F and add the perfume. Pour the molten wax carefully into the mold. Allow the candle to cool in a water bath.

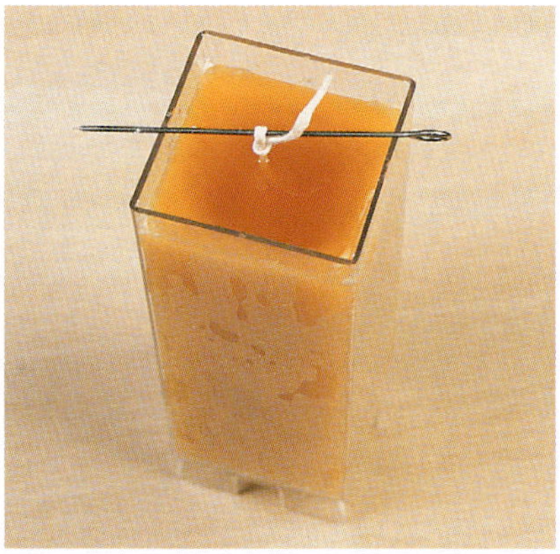

3 When the candle has set, reheat the wax to 200°F and fill the dip that has appeared around the wick, taking care that no wax runs down the sides of the candle. Allow to cool completely, then remove from the mold.

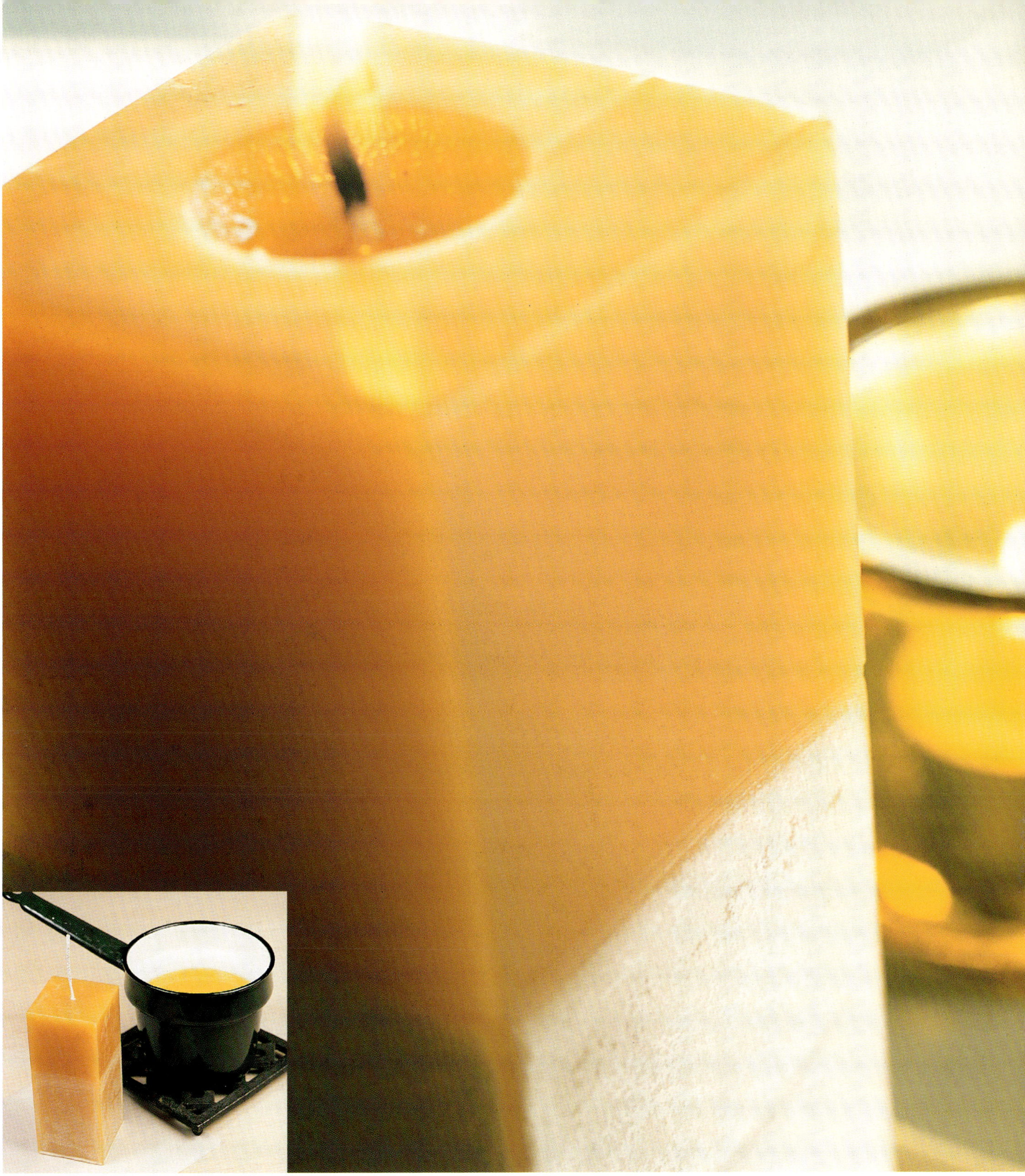

4 Melt enough crystalline dip in a pan to the depth you want to dip the candle to, and add a tiny amount of pigment. Heat to 180°F. Placing the pan level, hold the candle by the wick and dip it in the crystalline solution for 8–9 seconds, so the candle sits just briefly on the base of the pan. Remove from the pan and cool slowly.

Here a wax box forms the container for a candle that burns inside it, with the flame glowing through the box sides. Using an empty milk carton in waxed cardboard as a mold gives you professional results by taking a resourceful approach to candle making. Square molds of this size are not widely available, so it's satisfying to improvise with something from the supermarket shelf. The mold is filled with molten wax and left until the sides and base have set. When the molten wax inside is poured away, what remains is a perfectly formed box that can be used as the container for a scented candle. Only scent the actual candle; here rosewood and sandalwood make an exotic blend.

box candle

you will need:

6 oz. stearin
Wax dye
1 lb. 8 oz. paraffin wax
Prepared medium container wick
Wick sustainer
Approximately 1½ tsp. essential oil or candle perfume

MAKING THE CANDLE This wax "box" candle is made in a similar way to the bowl candle on page 68. You need enough wax to completely fill the mold, even though some of the wax inside the box will be poured out later. Prepare the mold by reinforcing the sides with pieces of cardboard held around the carton with masking tape—this prevents the sides from bowing outward when filled with hot wax, making a very effective mold. The wax is poured into the mold at a lower temperature to give a slightly textured effect. To give the box a smart crisp edge, run a hot iron over the rim. The candle cube measures 4 inches.

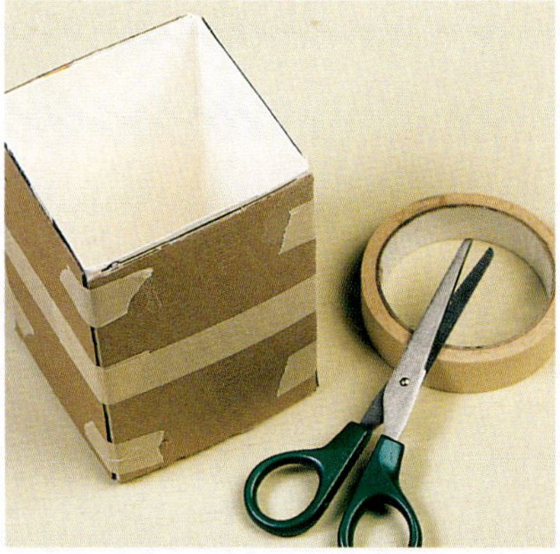

1 Reinforce the sides of the carton with pieces of cardboard held in place with masking tape. Make a mark inside the mold to show how high to fill it with wax so the finished depth is the same as the width of the box.

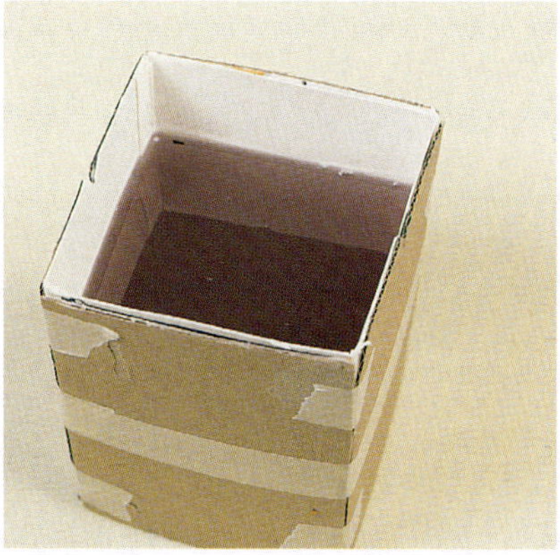

2 Melt the stearin and wax dye together, then add the paraffin wax and heat the mixture to 150°F. Pour the wax into the mold up to the mark. Allow to partly set.

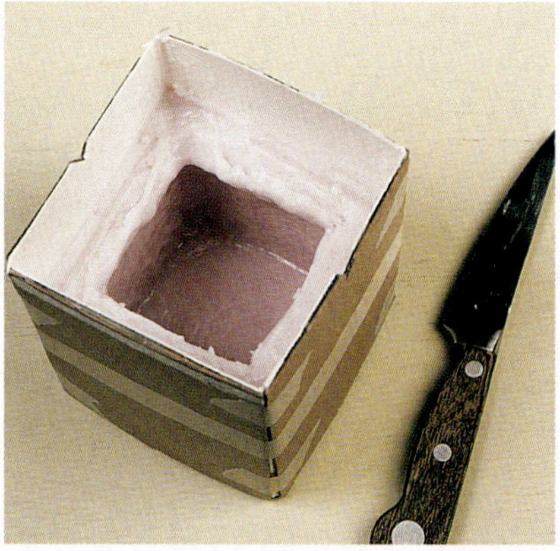

3 When sides have set to a thickness of approximately ½ inch, break the skin on the top of the wax and pour out the molten wax inside to leave a box with rough inner edges. Use a small knife to smooth the inside, then allow to cool completely.

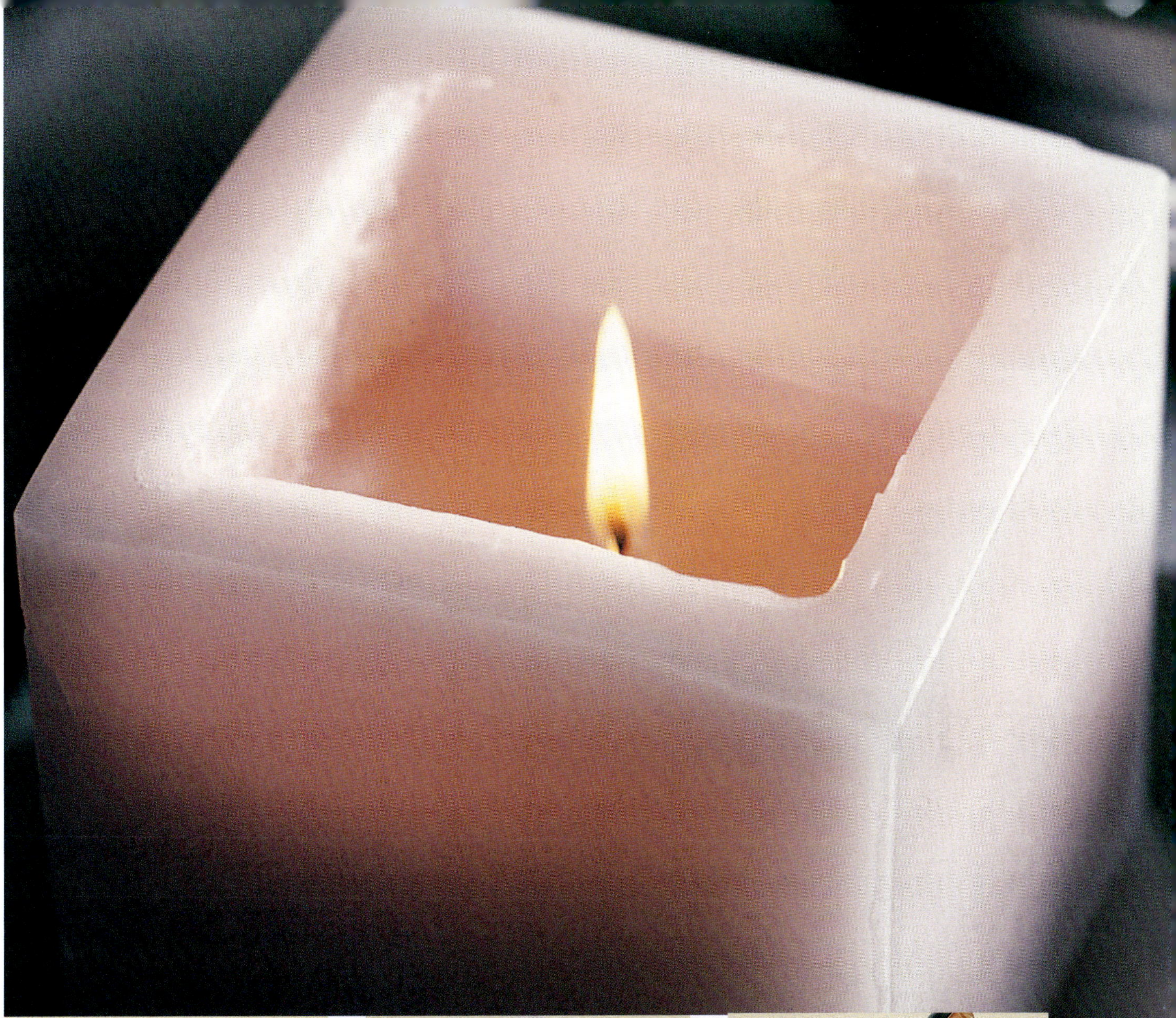

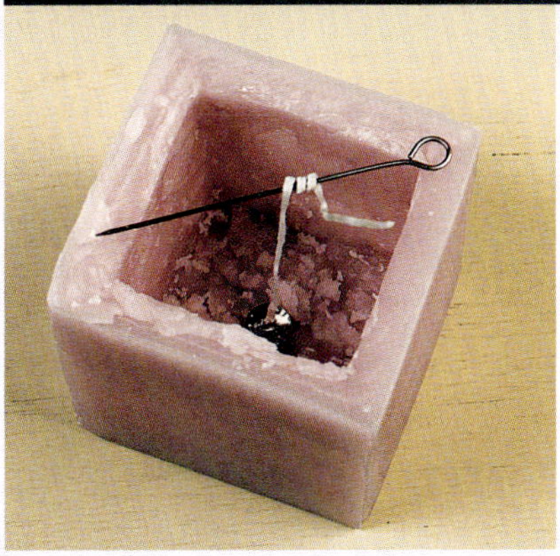

4 Tear the carton away to leave the wax box. Attach a wick sustainer to one end of the wick as before and place it centrally within the box, wrapping the excess wick around a wicking needle resting across the top.

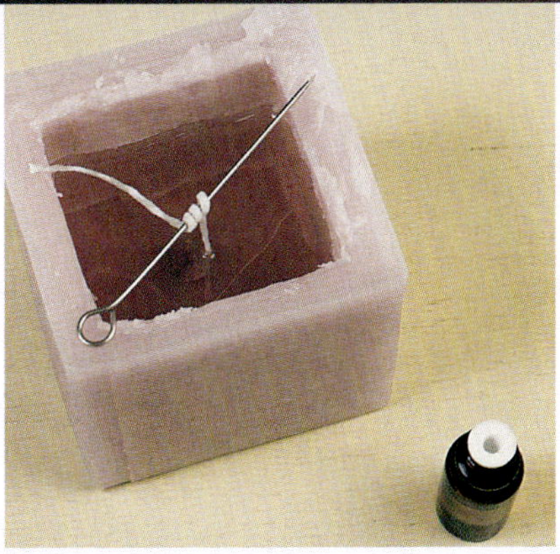

5 Reheat the wax to 150°F and add the perfume. Pour the scented wax into the box to within 1¼ inches of the rim. Allow it to set. If necessary, fill in the dip that forms as the wax sets.

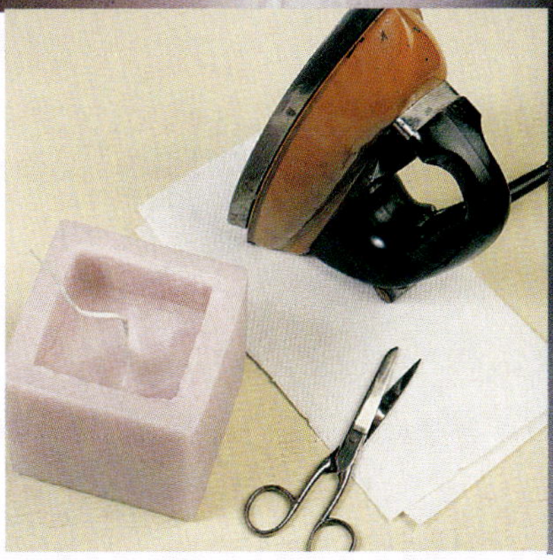

6 When the wax has completely set, trim the wick and flatten the top of the box sides by running a hot iron over the rim.

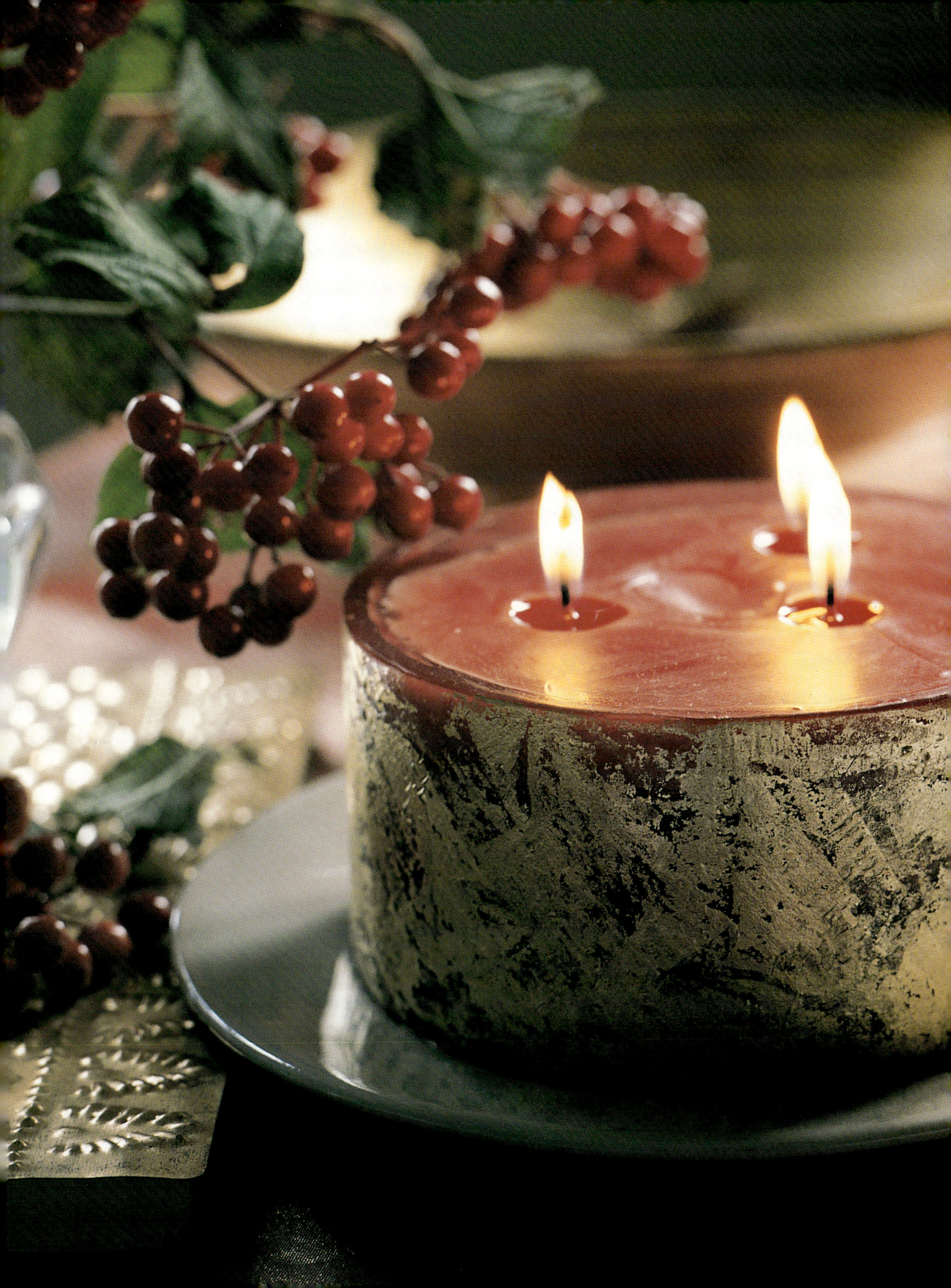

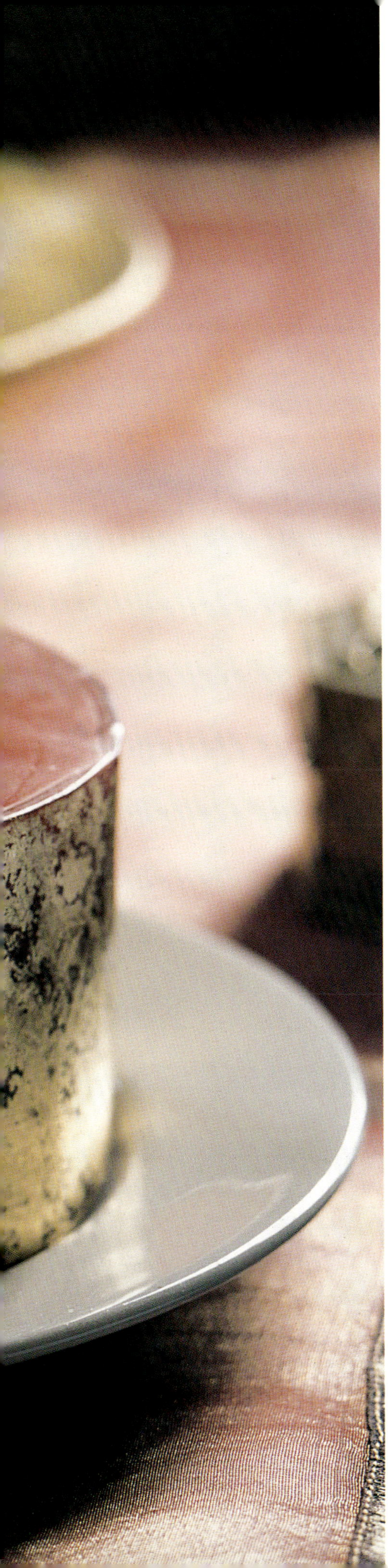

Gold leaf has a special quality and, when used to embellish a candle, looks stunning.

pillar candle

Using real gold leaf to decorate a candle gives a luxuriously lavish result. This can be bought in books containing several leaves of gold held flat between tissue paper backing sheets. The effect is easily achieved by placing the gold leaf with its backing sheet against the candle's surface so the gold touches the wax. Rub over the tissue with the back of a pair of scissors, applying a gentle pressure so the tissue paper doesn't tear. You will see the gold becoming fainter through the backing paper. Peel the paper away to leave the gilding on the wax surface. Scenting the candle with frankincense and myrrh creates a wonderfully spiritual ambience when the soothing, musty fragrances are combined.

In this project, the touch of luxury gives a true feeling of holiday, with the accents of real gold, and the frankincense and myrrh echoing the three gifts given at the very first Christmas. A deep red berry color adds opulence, while the aromas give a gentle uplifting feel to the ambience of a room. This candle is ideal as a table centerpiece, as the perfume is not too heavy to overpower the equally seasonal scents of the family Christmas meal.

you will need:

Prepared wick
Wick sustainers
Mold
6 oz. stearin
Wax dye
1 lb. 8 oz. paraffin wax
Approximately 1½ fl. oz. essential oil or candle perfume
Sheet of gold leaf

MAKING THE CANDLE A straight-sided glass tank vase makes an ideal mold for this wide, pillar candle, but be sure to check that your mold has no bumps inside as even the slightest inward curve will prevent the candle from coming out of the mold. Alternatively, use a plastic or tin paint can with straight sides. This candle is wide enough to accommodate three evenly spaced wicks. It measures 5 inches in diameter and 2¾ inches high.

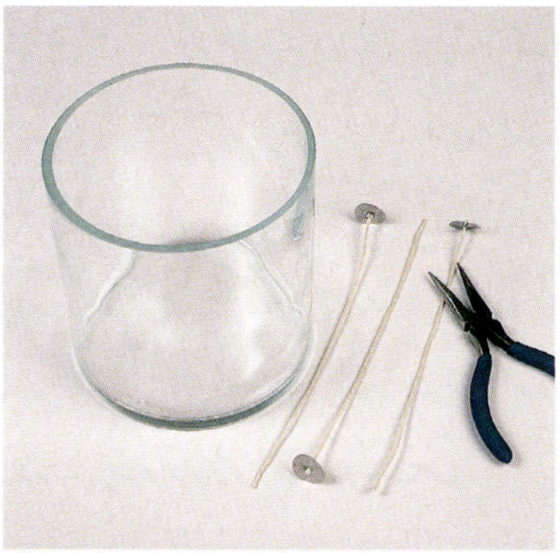

1 Cut three lengths of wick slightly longer than the depth of the mold. Attach wick sustainers to one end of each wick, closing the metal around the wick using pliers.

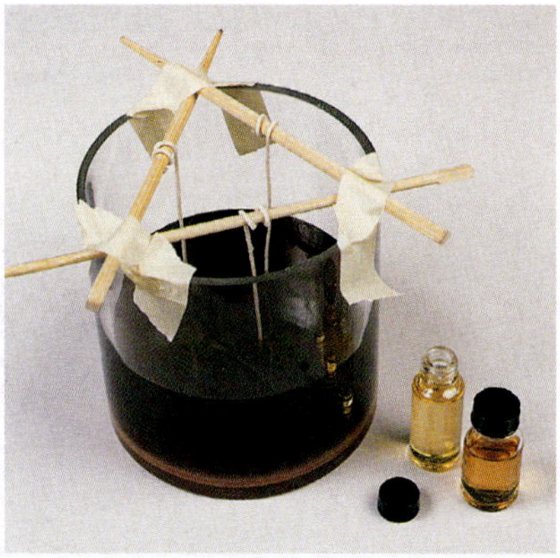

3 When the wax in the mold has slightly cooled, reheat the wax in the double boiler to 200°F, then add the perfume and pour the wax carefully into the mold to the required depth.

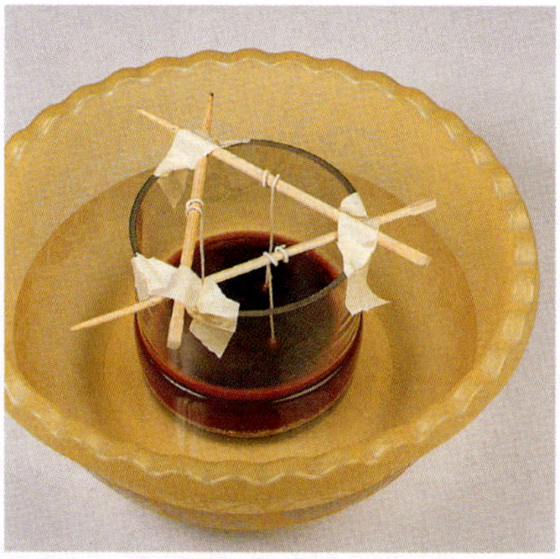

4 Place the mold in a water bath filled with cold water to cool the wax quickly and improve the surface of the candle. Allow to cool.

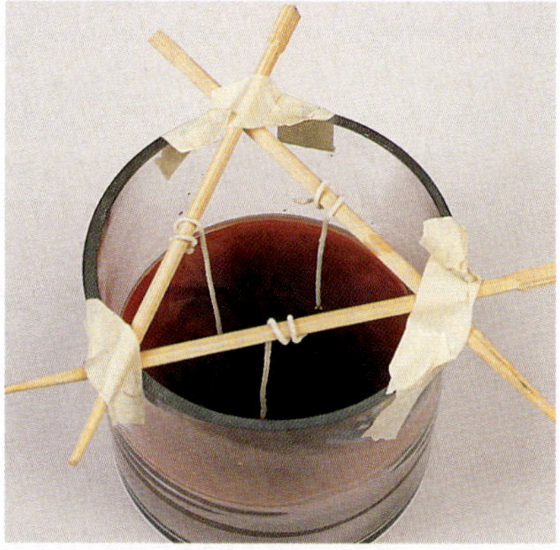

5 As the candle sets, the top shrinks down around the wicks, so reheat the wax and fill the dips carefully, making sure no wax runs down over the sides between the candle and the mold. Allow to set, then remove from the mold and trim the wicks.

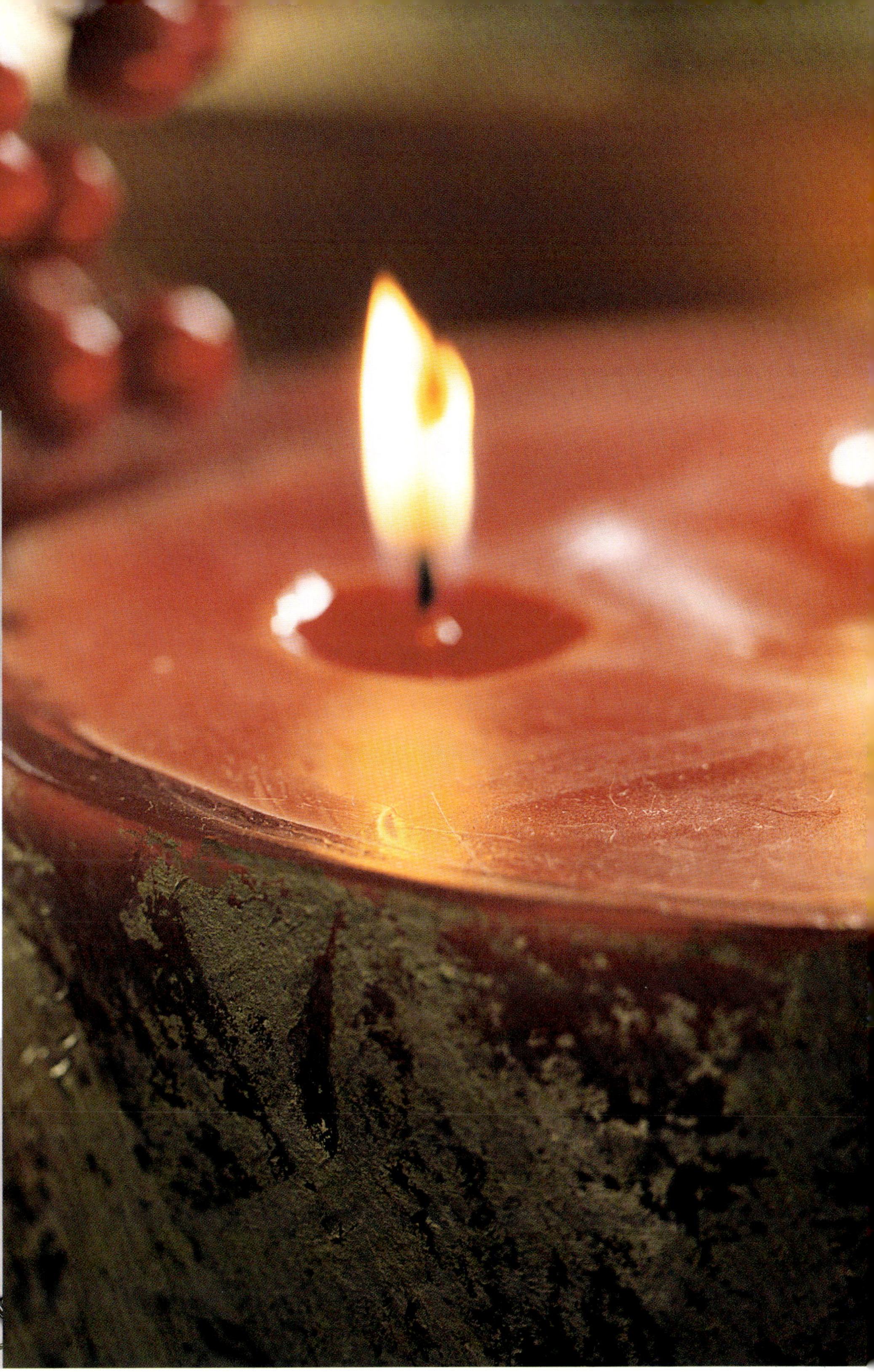

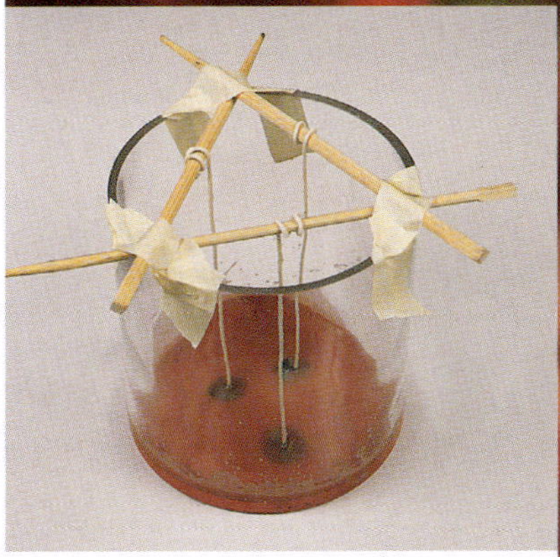

2 Place the wicks inside the mold with the sustainers on the base. Wind the excess wick around sticks or wicking needles resting across the rim. Melt the stearin and dye together, then add the paraffin wax. Heat to 200°F, then carefully pour a small amount into the mold.

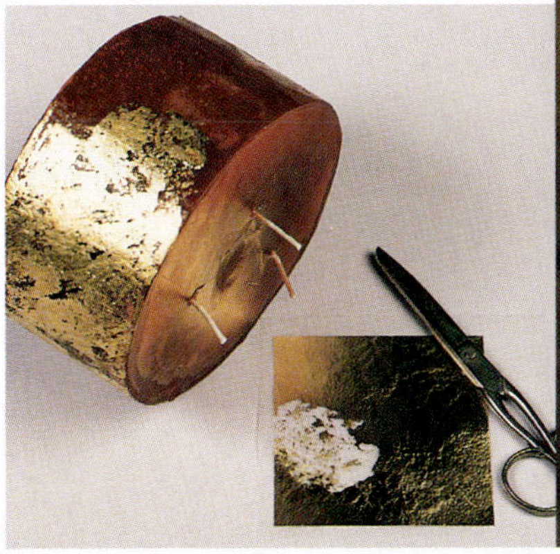

6 Place a sheet of gold leaf with paper backing carefully onto the candle. Gently rub the backing paper with the back of a pair of scissors. Remove the paper and reuse any bits of gold leaf left on the paper to fill in any gaps. Apply gold leaf all the way around the candle to complete the design.

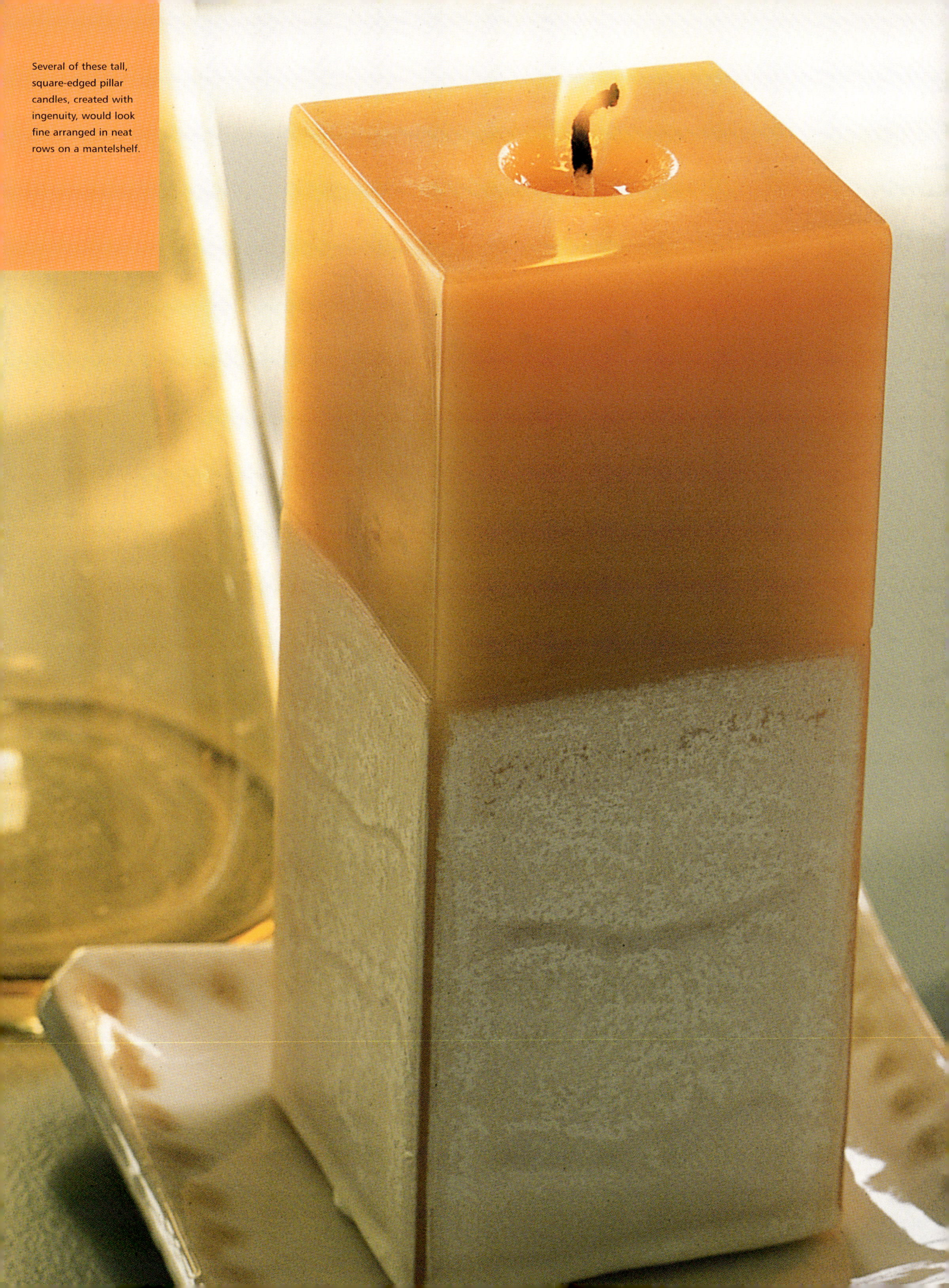

Several of these tall, square-edged pillar candles, created with ingenuity, would look fine arranged in neat rows on a mantelshelf.

WINTER COLORS

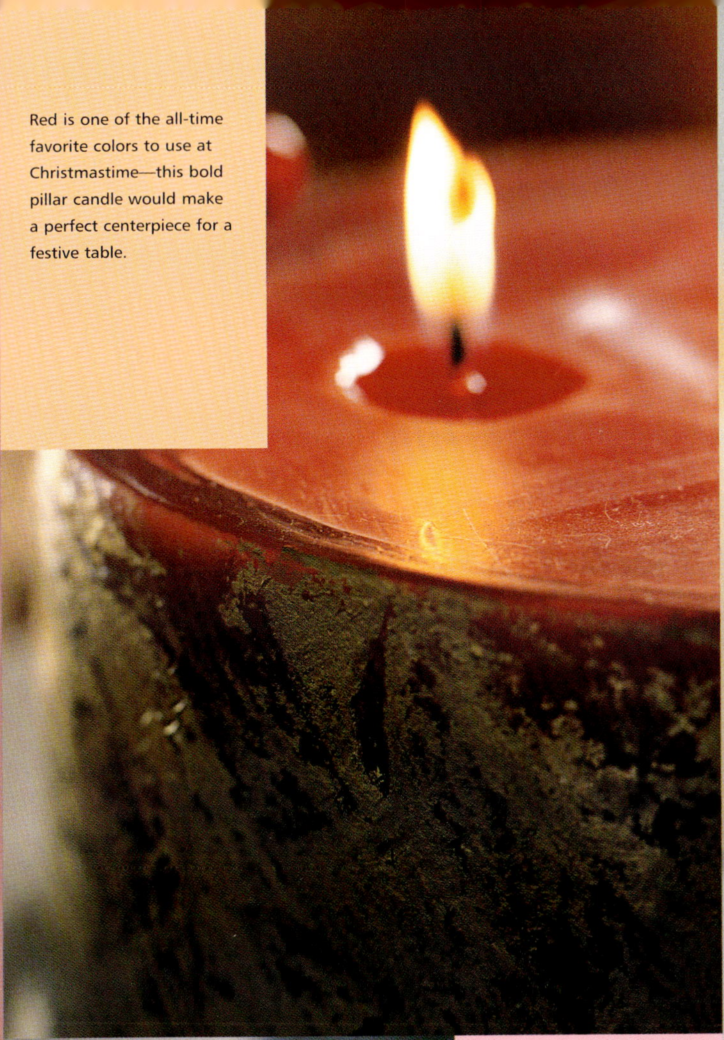

Red is one of the all-time favorite colors to use at Christmastime—this bold pillar candle would make a perfect centerpiece for a festive table.

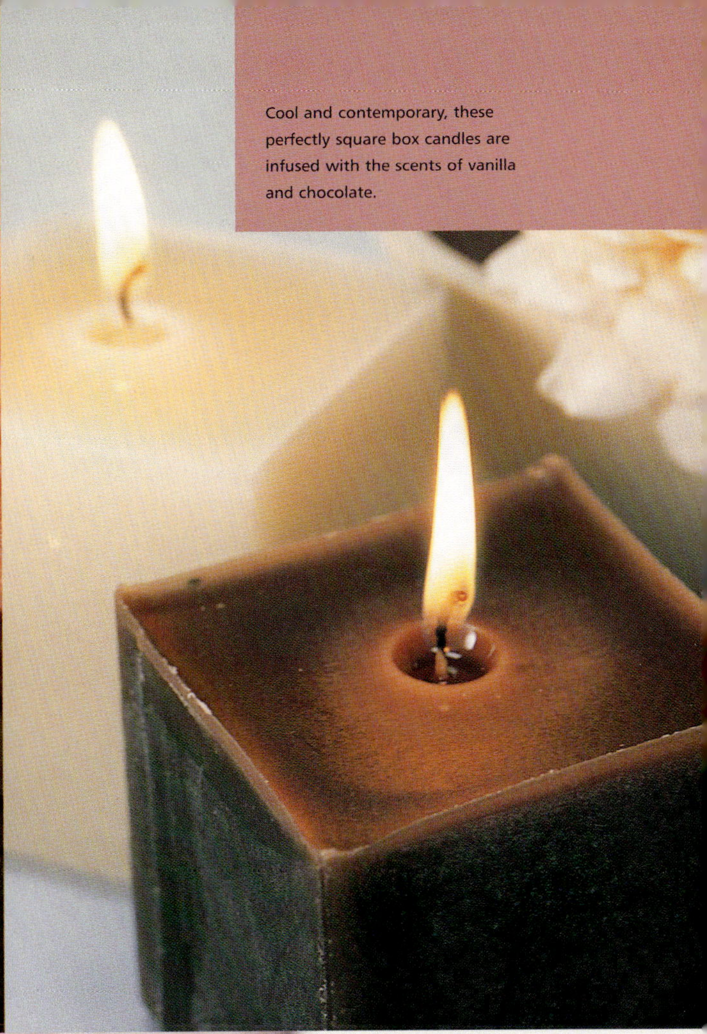

Cool and contemporary, these perfectly square box candles are infused with the scents of vanilla and chocolate.

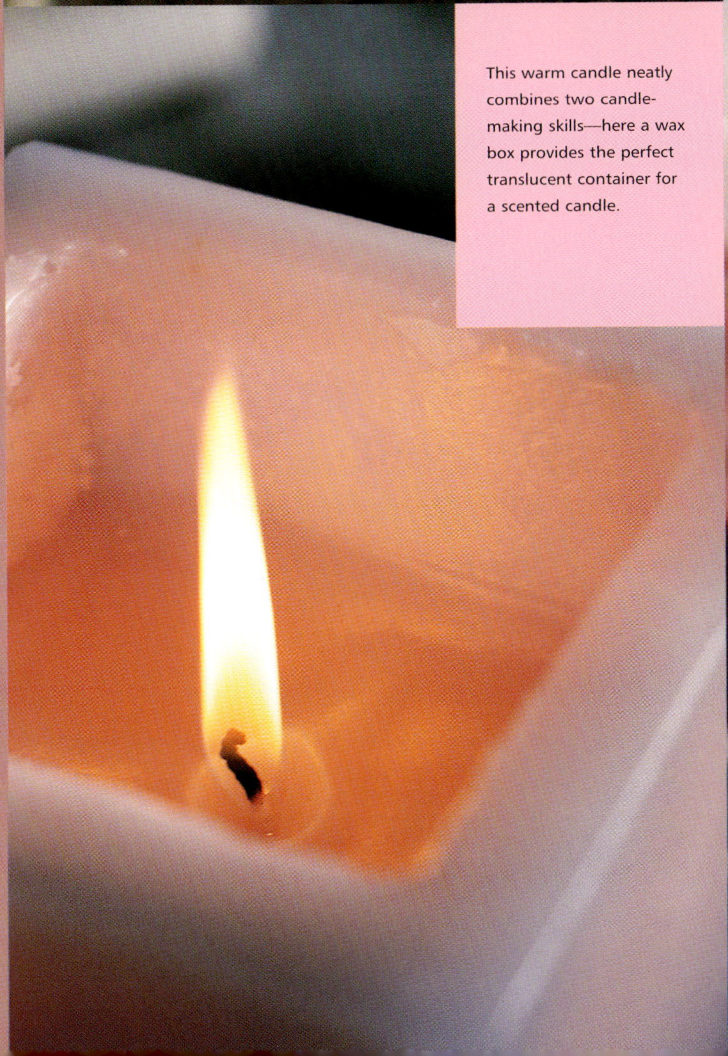

This warm candle neatly combines two candle-making skills—here a wax box provides the perfect translucent container for a scented candle.

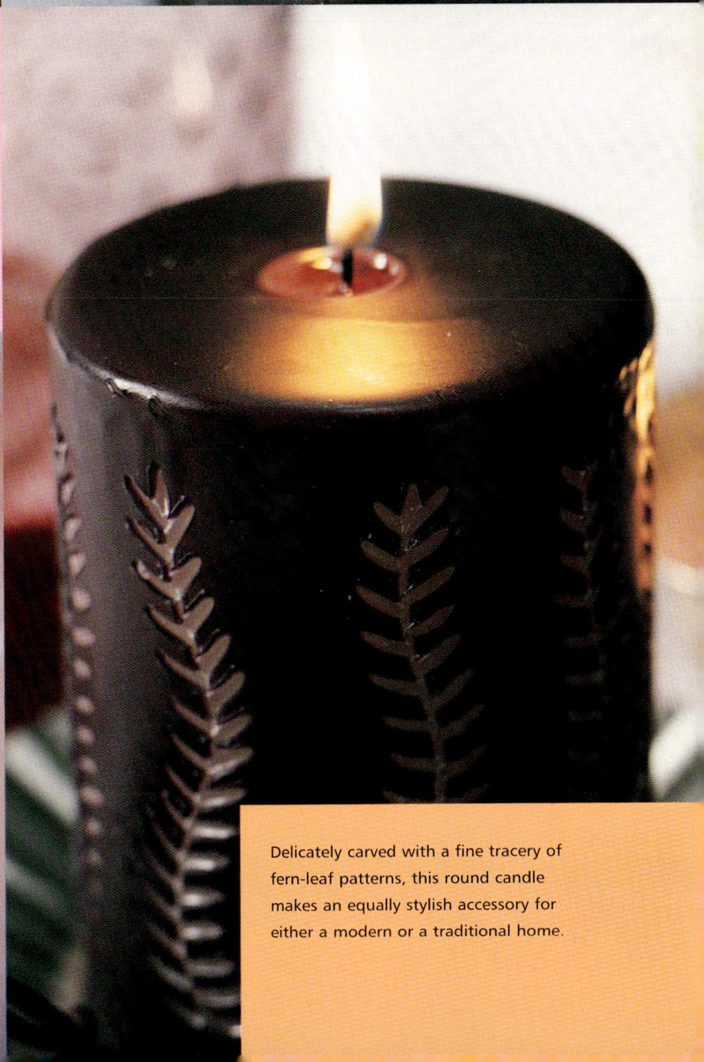

Delicately carved with a fine tracery of fern-leaf patterns, this round candle makes an equally stylish accessory for either a modern or a traditional home.

techniques

special equipment

dipping can Dipping cans come in various sizes and are a tall, cylindrical shape. They are used to make dipped candles and also for dipping candles in a final colored coating or to fix decoration to the candle surface. This specialist piece of equipment can be bought from a candle-making supplier, and is used by standing it in a pan of simmering water in the same way as a double boiler, with the water level as high up the sides as possible. It takes a fair amount of wax to fill a dipping can as the melted wax needs to be to the depth of the candle you are making or to become submerged by the wax when dipping. Use special dipping wax when making dipped candles.

double boiler As hot wax can become highly inflammable if it reaches too high a temperature, it is advisable to melt wax in the top of a double boiler. The pan should be made of stainless steel, aluminum, or be enamel-coated. If you do not have a double boiler, you can improvise by placing a smaller pan inside a larger one. Remember to check that the water in the bottom of the pan does not boil dry; keep filling it up if making candles over a long period. After pouring out the molten wax, wipe around the top of the pan with a dry paper towel to clean away the residue.

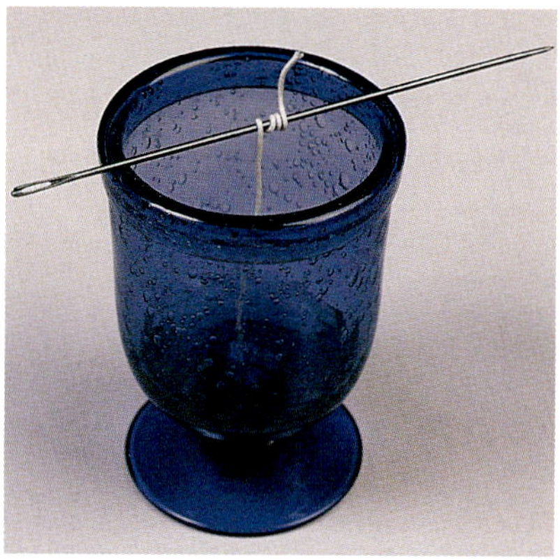

molds Candle molds can be made of glass, rubber, or plastic and are available in lots of shapes and sizes. Plastic ones tend to be less expensive than glass, and the rubber ones more ornate. Some molds for spherical and egg shapes come in two sections that separate across the middle. To make an unusual-shaped mold, use an oval glass vase or round tank vase, but be sure to choose one that gets wider toward the top so the candle will slide out without any problems, and check that there are no bumps inside that will make this difficult. Also, remember that unless the glass is pretty thick, it will crack from the heat. A tin paint can or clean plastic container with straight sides can be used to make a large cylinder candle with several wicks.

wax thermometer The temperature the wax is heated to alters the appearance of the surface on the finished candle, so it is important to have a special wax thermometer or a cooking thermometer that covers the range 100–225°F. To fill a container candle where the texture of the wax is unimportant, heat the wax to 160°F. For an interesting mottled and textured surface, the type found on the fashionable candles sold in interior design stores, the wax is poured quite cool and can be at a lower temperature, at around 150°F. For a clear, smooth, colored surface heat the wax to 200°F before pouring into the mold.

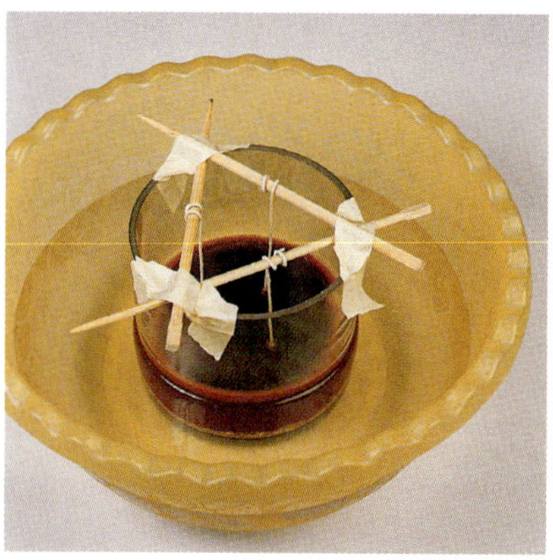

water bath Cooling the molten wax quickly helps to improve the surface appearance of the candle. To speed things up, place the mold of hot, molten wax in a bowl of cold water that comes up the sides of the mold to the level of the top of the wax. The mold will need to be weighed down with a heavy object on top to keep it steady.

hot iron To flatten candle bases, you can use an ordinary household iron heated to a warm setting. After use, be sure to clean the iron. Once you have finished, run the iron along newspaper while it is still warm to clean it and remove any excess wax.

CHOOSING THE WICK

Wicks come in various sizes and should be chosen to suit the size of your mold or container. If the wick is too small, the flame will be too small. A small wick may also cause the candle to drip or may be extinguished in a pool of molten wax. Wicks should be kept trimmed to ½–1 inch in length. They are usually made of braided cotton and come in sizes ranging from ½ inch–4 inches in ½-inch gradations. Match the wick size to the diameter of the candle: you would need a 1-inch wick for a candle the same diameter. Special container wicks have a central core running through them, which helps to support the wick as the surrounding wax gets hot and molten. Extinguish container candles by using a metal object to push the wick into the surrounding pool of wax to drown the flame, then pulling the wick upright again so it is primed and ready for next time. If the candle is blown out the wick may smolder and disappear down into the wax surface, thus making it difficult to relight. When a candle is burned, keep the wick trimmed to ⅛–¼-inch high at all times.

PRIMING THE WICK

All wicks need to be primed except when making dipped candles or when using rubber molds. To prime the wick, melt a little paraffin wax in a double boiler and let the wick soak in it for a few minutes so it becomes coated. Remove the wick from the wax and straighten, leaving it to dry on a baking sheet.

DYEING THE WAX

Dyeing wax is similar to mixing paints but it is more difficult to gauge accurately as molten wax often bears absolutely no resemblance to the color it will be when set. Wax dye comes in flat disks of highly concentrated color that can be cut into segments. It is usually melted with the stearin before adding the paraffin wax. Finely ground candle pigment can also be used in the same way and is used instead of wax dye when making gel candles. To get an accurate idea of what the final color will be, drop a small pool of molten wax onto a baking sheet and let it set. When mixing together leftover colored wax and recycling the ends of candles, only mix colors within a particular shade rather than lots of different contrasting colors, to prevent the new color from ending up a dirty, muddy brown. The amount of stearin in the candle improves the vibrancy of the color and should account for between 10 and 30 percent of the volume of the candle.

PERFUME SAFETY AND ADDING SCENT

You can add 2–5 percent of perfume to a wax candle, so adjust the amount to suit your own taste, making the candle as subtle or powerful as you like. The perfume can lower the flash point of the wax—the temperature at which it becomes flammable—so take extreme care when heating wax to higher temperatures, and never add more than 5 percent perfume. Wax perfumes are made specifically for this purpose with safety in mind. Gel candles burn at higher temperatures than wax candles, so when you are making gel candles, take particular care when scenting with essential oils; never use more than 2 percent essential oil in the project, and always follow the instructions. When using essential oils in all projects follow the tests shown on page 8 to check their suitability.

HOW MUCH WAX?

To work out the quantity of wax you will need to fill your container or mold, fill it with water and measure the amount it takes. Substitute 3 oz. wax for every 3½ fl. oz. of liquid, adding a little bit extra for luck.

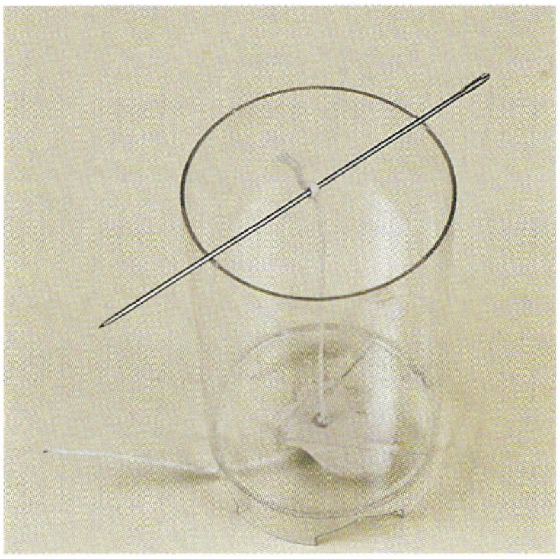

MOLDED CANDLES

Special molds bought from craft stores usually make the candle upside down, so its top will be in the base of the mold. The advantage of this is that the top of the candle will be perfectly smooth and might have a slightly raised, pointed top. Candles made the other way up, so the top of the candle is formed by the last wax poured into the mold, are much harder to make with a smooth surface. As the wax sets and shrinks, cavities form around the wicks and they need to be filled with more wax. If the candle top is uneven, you can smooth it out with a hot iron afterward.

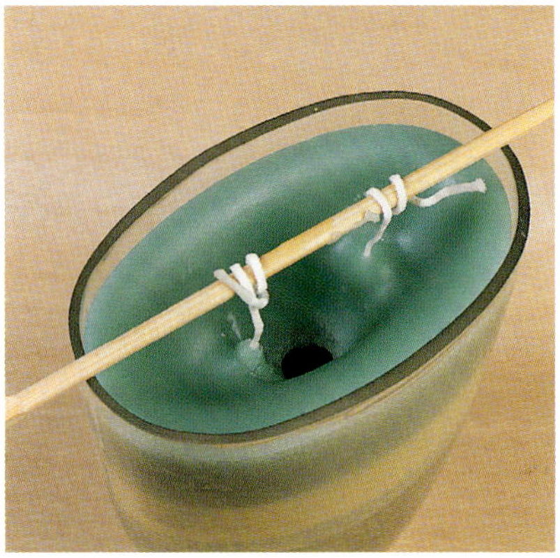

FILLING UP

With store-bought molds the wick usually threads through a hole in the base which needs to be sealed and secured with mold sealant. The other end of the wick needs to be held tightly through the mold by tying it to a wicking needle held across the rim. Stearin is added to the wax to improve the appearance of the candle and works as a shrinking agent so the candle comes out of the mold easily. (When using a rubber mold, Vybar is used instead of stearin, as this can harm the rubber.) The stearin, dye, and paraffin wax are heated together to the required temperature and then poured into the mold. For the best results, use a water bath to cool the wax quickly. Fill the cavity around the wick with more wax and allow to set.

When making the candle in a makeshift mold, it is necessary to make holes in the base or, alternatively, make the candle the right way up and set up the wicks using wick sustainers that will hold the wicks in place.

DIPPED CANDLES

Dipped candles are made in pairs. A long length of wick held in the middle is dipped repeatedly in molten wax, building up the shape of the candle layer by layer. The core of the candle can be made in plain white wax, which is then given a final dip in colored wax. Heat the wax to 160°F in a dipping can sitting in a pan of water, holding a length of wick in the center, and prime the wick by dipping both ends in the wax and soaking them for 1 minute; then remove and hang up to dry. While dipping, the two candles are strangely drawn together and need to be kept separate and hung up between dips so they do not touch each other as the wax sets. When the wicks are cool, dip them again in the wax, submerging them for 3 seconds then allowing them to cool for 1–4 minutes between dips, depending on the room temperature. Repeat the process until the candle is the required thickness. Finally, dip a few times, as before, in colored wax heated to 180°F to give a smooth, even surface. Leave the candles to set, level the candle bases with a hot iron, and separate the wicks. After you have finished with the iron, run it along newspaper while it is still warm to clean it and remove any excess wax. Allow them to cool for at least 1 hour before burning. Dipping candles is the least suitable method of making scented candles, as standing over a can of hot, scented wax could become quite nauseating, resulting in a headache and a lifelong aversion to that particular scent, so use unscented wax to form the shape, then spoon over a few layers of hot scented wax before the final colored dipping.

SAFETY GUIDELINES: USING CANDLES

If you are giving candles as gifts, be sure to make a label that passes on these safety guidelines to the recipient as well as always acting on them yourself. Never leave lighted candles unattended or place them on unsteady surfaces or in a drafty place. Always place candles on stands or dishes. Handle hot wax with extreme care and, while candle making, keep pan handles turned away from people or anywhere where they might be knocked over. Never place lit candles close to walls, textiles, or any other material that could become hazardous, and keep candles away from children and pets. Remember that as they burn, candles use up oxygen in the room and give off lots of heat, so watch that the calming and warming atmosphere they can create doesn't send you to sleep. Don't allow the candle to burn for more than 3 hours or to burn down to the bottom of the container. As the candle burns, keep the wick trimmed to ⅛–¼-inch high at all times. If you make a candle with free-floating elements in it, remove the pieces as the candle burns down. Use your common sense and exercise caution. See the warning on page 4.

glossary

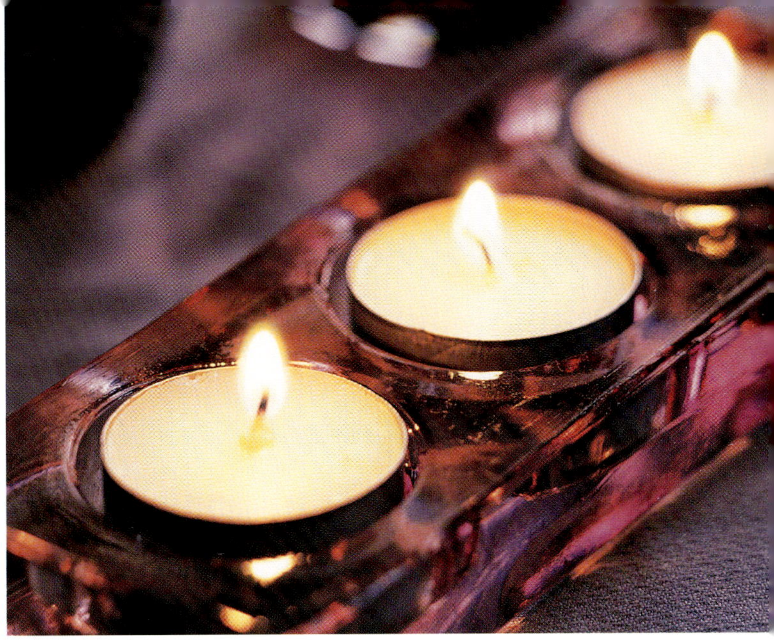

PARAFFIN WAX

This is the basic wax used for candle making. It is a colorless, odorless by-product of oil refining. It is generally sold as beads that melt at a temperature of 105–160°F. Stearin (see below) is often added when making molded candles, and paraffin wax can be purchased with the stearin already included.

BEESWAX

Beeswax is a completely natural product found in beehives as part of the honeycomb surrounding the honey. It is expensive but has a wonderful scent and produces candles with a longer burning time and clear, white flames. It comes in natural shades, from pale cream to pale honey brown. If more than 10 percent of beeswax is used in a molded candle, you may need to apply a releasing agent to the mold, as it has a sticky quality.

DIP-AND-CARVE WAX

This is a blend of waxes specially formulated so it can be carved without splintering. It has a particularly malleable quality and comes in solid slabs.

CANDLE GEL

Gel for candle making is a clear material that has become popular in recent years for container candles. It is easy to work with as you simply melt the gel and pour it in. Its transparent quality makes it possible to embed flowers and objects in the candle so they show through. When set, the gel peels off surfaces easily.

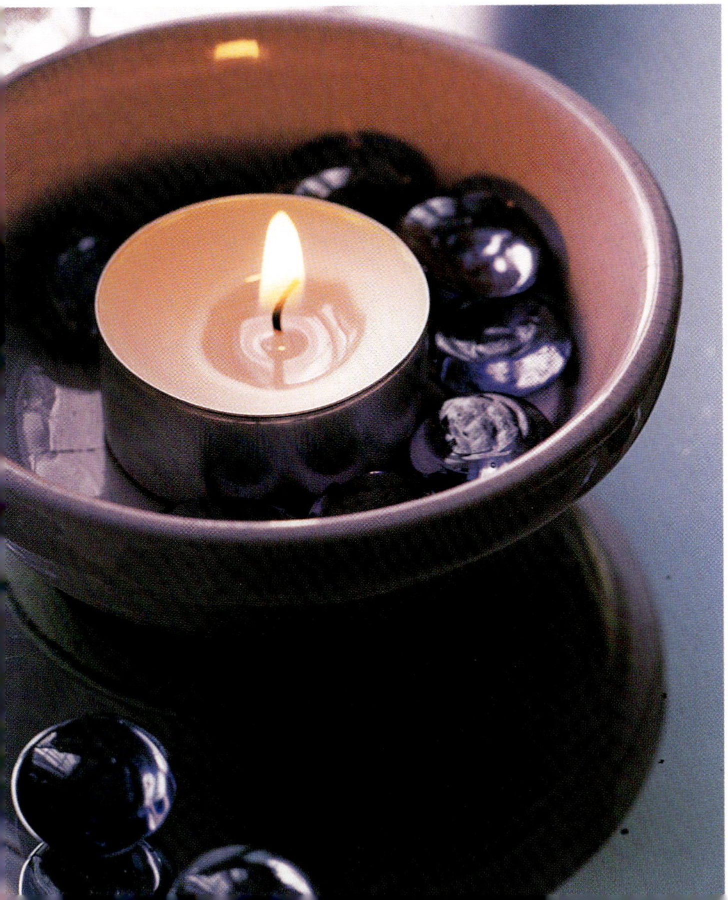

STEARIN

This is used as an additive to paraffin wax to increase its shrinking abilities so it releases easily from a mold. It also improves the quality of a candle by helping to stop any drips when burning and gives a quality finish to the wax. As a rule, use between 10 and 20 percent of stearin to paraffin wax.

VYBAR

Vybar is used as an additive to paraffin wax in much the same way as stearin. It improves the burning time and the color of the wax. When using rubber molds, use Vybar instead of stearin, which rots the rubber.

CRYSTALLINE DIP

This decorative dip is a kind of wax made from modified stearic acid. It handles like wax but dries with an interesting mottled effect. One dip of 8–9 seconds is sufficient to create the effect on the surface of a candle, and the longer it takes to dry, the more effective the texture will be.

WAX GLUE

This is a soft, sticky wax available in solid form. It is used to glue wax surfaces together or to apply decoration, such as dried flowers or foil shapes, to the sides of candles.

MOLD SEAL

This is a reuseable putty used to seal holes in molds to make them watertight and prevent wax from leaking out. Make sure no residue remains on the wick or it might make lighting the candle problematic.

WICK SUSTAINERS

These are metal disks used to anchor the wick in container candles. Push one end of the wick through the sustainer and pinch the metal closed with pliers to hold it tightly in place. The sustainer sits on the bottom of the container.

WICKING NEEDLES

Wicking needles are used to hold the wicks in place and rest across the rim of the mold. Wick can be wrapped around the needle or the needle can be pushed through the wick to hold it secure. Use chopsticks or pencils for the same purpose instead.

index

suppliers

Candles and Supplies.com
301 S. 3rd St. (Rt. 309)
Coopersburg, PA 18036
Tel: (610) 282–5522
www.candlesandsupplies.com

Jo-Ann Fabric & Crafts
841 Apollo St., Suite 350
El Segundo, CA 90245
Tel: (888) 739–4120
www.joann.com

Michaels
8000 Bent Branch Dr.
Irving, TX 75063
Tel: (800) Michaels
www.michaels.com

MisterArt.com
913 Willard St.
Houston, TX 77006
Tel: (866) MR–ART–11
www.misterart.com

The Candlewic Company
825 Easton Road
Doylestown, PA 18901
Tel: (215) 230–3601
Fax: (215) 230–3606
www.candlewic.com

U.K. & European stockists:

Candle Makers Supplies
28 Blythe Road,
London W14 0HA
Tel: (01144) 020 7602 4031
www.candlemakers.co.uk

G Baldwin & Co
171/173 Walworth Road
London SE17 1RW
Tel: (01144) 020 7703 5550

author's acknowledgments

I would particularly like to thank David Constable from Candle Makers Supplies, who with over thirty years of candle-making experience so generously shared his hard-earned knowledge with me, contributed materials as well as the rose floating candles (p. 40), the embossed candle (p. 56), and the 1960s candle (p. 22) projects. Also, thanks are due to Graham Morgan from Candle Makers Supplies for making the 1960s candle and getting it to me just in the nick of time. Thanks to Deborah Schneebeli-Morrell for coming over one afternoon and completing the carved candle (p. 76) as well as trying to sort me out—no chance! And to Emma Hardy for help with styling and putting up with me wittering on. Finally, a big thank you to everyone at Cico: Cindy Richards and Georgina Harris for being so encouraging and Christine Wood, who has done such a fabulous job designing the book.